A *must-read* for parents of all deaf children
and those interested in the deaf. Complete
insight on everything one should know about
residential deaf schools and the
culturally deaf community's way of life.

A culturally deaf writer's expose' of the deaf
"culture," with information the deaf
community does not want publicly revealed.

A first-hand report from a writer educated at a
residential deaf school with a disclosure of
many shocking circumstances
surrounding residential deaf schools.

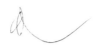

A CHILD SACRIFICED

The author would like thank all the culturally deaf persons who contributed towards an accurate portrayal of the deaf community for this book. Special notes of appreciation goes to Bob Fowler, the deaf community's leading book expert, to Kay Morris, for her touch on the finishing details and to Valerie Jo, for all her patience.

A CHILD SACRIFICED
TO THE DEAF CULTURE

TOM BERTLING

KODIAK MEDIA GROUP
WILSONVILLE, OREGON

A CHILD SACRIFICED

First edition published 1994

10 9 8 7 6 5 4 3 2 1

For further information contact: KODIAK MEDIA GROUP, P.O. Box 1029-B, Wilsonville, Oregon 97070

SAN: 297-9993

ISBN 0-9637813-4-0

U.S. Library of Congress Catalog Card Number 93-79790

PUBLISHER'S CATALOGING IN PUBLICATION DATA
Bertling, Tom
A child sacrificed to the deaf culture.
  Bibliography and index.
  1. Deafness-children. 2. Deaf culture. 3. Parents of handicapped children. 4. Deaf education-schools. I Title.

This publication was produced in the State of Oregon.

CONTENTS

A CHILD SACRIFICED

*There is very little agreement among all the factors involved with the education of the deaf child. Parents of deaf children must explore all possibilities, then weigh all the advantages against the disadvantages to make the best decision for **their** child. Parents should also be wary of proponents of methods of educating the deaf that seem to be mostly criticism of other methods.*

*Some of the names, places, titles, and genders may have been changed or deleted to protect the privacy of people involved in my experiences. It is **not my intent to identify or ridicule** anyone in this book, but rather to relate life in the deaf culture and the deaf school as it happened to me.*

This author's views are based upon personal experiences and opinions and does not pretend to be the final and absolute authority on this subject matter.

FOREWORD
A Different Perspective

The primary objective of this book is to promote awareness in the mainstream hearing society of the culturally deaf world, as well as those living in it, of its unspoken shortcomings. Most notably, and the most disappointing, is the failure of the culture to produce citizens who are, by and large, *contributors to society.*

By this, I am referring to an deaf adult being able to earn an income to support himself, his family, and by the way of being a taxpayer, to support the continual existence of our society.

I feel that a deaf person can be a contributor to society at a level equal to the rest of the hearing society. While many do succeed at this, however, I feel many of the leaders of the deaf culture have placed an importance of trying to *preserve the deaf culture* over the best interest of its members and our society in general.

The residential school for the deaf is virtually the deaf culture's only avenue to ensure the culture thrives. Without residential deaf schools, the deaf culture as it exists today would be profoundly different, and this is what the leaders of the deaf culture fear

A CHILD SACRIFICED

While the residential school for the deaf excels at breeding a deaf culture, it seems to fail at preparing a deaf person to live in the mainstream hearing world. Large numbers of deaf adults are under educated, often unwilling, or simply unable to cope with life outside the deaf culture after leaving the segregated nature of a residential deaf school.

Confused parents of deaf children are often convinced by these deaf leaders to send their child to a residential deaf school without grasping the true impact the experience will have on him. They are also unaware of possible ulterior motives.

Leaders of the culturally deaf combat threats to their existence by gaining influence over decisions regarding the future of deaf children. They have stated, because they are deaf, that they should be consulted as experts, before doctors, educators, or school administrators, over the education of a deaf child.

Obviously, some input from the culturally deaf is necessary. However, we must keep in mind, new or different methods of teaching, new medical advancements and treatments taking the deaf child out of the deaf community environment is something they must prevent.

Parents should cast a cautious eye towards anyone wanting to *sacrifice a deaf child towards preserving a culture.*

It is not my intent to condemn the culturally deaf way of life or belittle its importance, but rather to bring it to reality for those uninitiated, by looking at the deaf culture from a different perspective, the view from inside looking out.

This is a fresh perspective, an examination of a residential school for the deaf, a culture and a way of life by someone living it. I intend to open windows into the deaf world that are not normally open to those on the outside.

While much has been written and debated over the nuts and bolts of educating the deaf, the deaf culture and deafness itself, this is a revealing· experience of *living the culturally deaf way of life*.

I do not pretend to be an educator of the deaf nor to have the last word on deaf education, but speak from the *experience of being educated by the culturally deaf favored method of education*. That is being educated at a residential school for the deaf where classes are taught in sign language, mostly using ASL (American Sign Language).

Published non-biased views of the culturally deaf world by the people who live the culturally deaf life is almost non-existent. Few are in a position to get their views published. Material published on the deaf culture, by the culturally deaf, is often biased towards a continual existence of the culture. By being employed, or having their field of expertise dependent on a deaf culture, the writers are not likely to put their jobs and livelihood in jeopardy.

In some cases, this is carried to an extreme. Some deaf writers for large and widely read deaf newspapers regularly write biased and substanceless articles, (with some exceptions) being more of a "rally cry for the deaf cause" seemingly, than anything else. It is disturbing to me because too many people (hearing or deaf) are exposed to these biased views on the deaf culture. Means to obtain a balanced view is not readily available.

An alternative is the works of hearing authors who have done research into the deaf culture, however they often get views presented by the same people dependent on the deaf culture for their existence. It is also difficult to get a true deaf "flavor" to the material.

I am not dependent on the deaf culture for employment, nor am I a writer as a profession. I have no financial need to write this book. Only the desire for change in the deaf culture has prompted me to write this on behalf of myself and the numerous others who feel the same way but because of the "unwritten rules" of the deaf culture, they remain silent in order to continue living in the deaf community.

When I make references to the "deaf culture" (also, the deaf community, the deaf world, the culturally deaf), it is directed to a select group of deaf people that primarily communicate in ASL. They also often have in common an education at a residential type school for the deaf. This does not include deaf individuals educated at oral-method facilities or related methods, nor includes deaf people who consider themselves "hard of hearing" and function primarily in the hearing society without ever being touched by the deaf culture.

I may at this time point out that sign language itself has nothing to do with the judgment I pass on the deaf culture. While it is convenient for the deaf culture to use ASL as a pedestal to base their culture upon, the bottom line is that most deaf adults will or should learn some form of sign language. The ability to have unrestricted communication at least with some people, is necessary sometimes to preserve sanity and prevent feelings of isolation. However, we must look at the deaf community's claim of an existence of a "culture" with some skepticism as they seem to base it upon ASL being the "natural" language of the deaf, not English. To disregard or diminish the language of the rest of our society cannot possibly benefit our deaf children.

A CHILD SACRIFICED

Leaders of the deaf community, when referred to by me, are culturally deaf people who through either appointment by others or elected outright to positions in which they can create changes within the deaf community. These are also esteemed members of the deaf community not having any official position. They could be officers of deaf organizations, including social, educational, fraternal associations, deaf educators, school and college administrators, and deaf people in social, community, and vocational services and agencies.

When I refer to deaf leaders unfavorably, I don't necessarily mean all of them. There are *many leaders who are good,* but often take the position of reflecting the attitudes of the deaf community that put them in power. Their actions and views might not necessarily be their own.

Keep in mind, some circumstances that might have been true at one time may no longer be true at this writing, but have been included as a historical content to accurately portray this subject.

The culturally deaf often capitalize the "d" in deaf to identify the person as being culturally deaf and as a sign of respect for them. Lower case is used to describe the non-culturally deaf. This is not standard English protocol and I see no need to deviate from it. Aside from confusing readers in the hearing society, it is a subtle method of persuasion, one of the existence of a deaf culture. [1]

My qualifications to being a member of the culturally deaf community are, a very severe hearing loss at age 5, educated in a state residential school for the deaf from 4th grade to graduation, usage of ASL for 25 years, having a deaf parent, grandparents, siblings and many other relatives, all fluent in ASL, deaf friends, membership and participation in deaf organizations.

I feel the dimension of *having lived the deaf culture experience* overshadows all the academic honors one may have to be a qualified authority on the deaf culture. This is a view shared by a highly respected and regarded leader of the deaf community who penned his own book on the deaf culture. 2

This book is sure to draw criticism and opposition from many leaders of the deaf community. Perhaps it may open eyes towards new thinking and changes within the deaf community to benefit them and the society in which we all live. At the very least, it will add a new source to balance knowledge of the deaf culture.

Readers should have concern of the happenings in the deaf culture. Some for being parents of deaf children, others for knowing or having an interest in the deaf. For most readers, as concerned citizens in our society, for *virtually every aspect of the deaf culture is subsidized by our tax dollars.*

Although my book will often reflect on the shortcomings in the deaf community, this should not be construed as approval of the current and past treatment of the deaf by the hearing society. *The hearing injustices towards the deaf could fill another book* and is beyond the subject matter at hand.

A CHILD SACRIFICED

CHAPTER ONE
A CHILDHOOD'S END

The first year at the deaf school, I was ten years old in the fourth grade. My first class of the day was leather shop. The classroom was at the far end of the institution grounds facing one of the main streets through town. I spent much time in the storage room looking out the window at the activity across the street. There were businesses plus a public elementary school much like the one I had gone to before being sent here.

The street became a symbol of the stark reality of where I was and the "outside world" I had once belonged. I would watch the grade school kids walk to school in the playful and happy manner I had done myself once upon a time. I have never felt as sad as I did watching the world go on without me.

As the months went by, I found it easier to fight back the tears as I looked out the storeroom window, but forever etched in my mind are those dark dreary November mornings that my childhood came to an end.

A few months earlier, on the first morning of the new school year at the state deaf school, all the children gathered in the auditorium for assignment to teachers and classes. The names of the students were called in sign language; then assigned to a teacher and reported to class.

Not having any knowledge of sign language, I sat through the whole process, not knowing if my name was called, not to mention the bewilderment of not being sure of what was going on and what might eventually happen to me. On top of all that, I was dealing with a sense of abandonment for being sent here. I felt I was being punished for not hearing better when I was in the public school.

After nearly everybody had finally dispersed did somebody had concern for me. I was made to wait in a foyer for quite a while until there was enough finger pointing done at me and a flurry of conversations in sign language giving me the impression of them being mystified about what to do with me.

Then somebody lead me from the intermediate school building and started to walk me to a different building where the first through third grades were taught. I would have entered fifth grade had I remained in public school and now here I was being lead to the primary school.

I remember vividly wondering what I might have done wrong to be headed towards this fate. Was it because I did not see my name being fingerspelled out? Did I look at somebody wrong? I did not know the proper way for a deaf person to behave and remember thinking that I must have done something wrong.

The walk to the school building seemed to take years. With an unexplained ominous future looming ahead, I was reliving what was a happy childhood prior to being sent here. All the scenes were replaying as I walked. It seemed slowly what was my life was now becoming someone else's. Although I did not know it at the time, for the rest of my time at this deaf school, things felt somewhat the same as one would describe as being transcendental. I would from then on be present but mentally distanced as a way to cope.

I was told to sit in a chair in the hall outside the administration office apparently used for disciplinary purposes. Drawing stares and mockery by ignorant students unaware of my plight, I became embarrassed and angry for not knowing what was happening to me.

I dared not ask anybody in fear of making another mistake. I felt hurt over the loss of my old life and was disturbed by not knowing what I had done, resulting in being placed in this deaf school.

It was after lunch before the primary school principal lead me to my new classroom and told me it was the second grade as I entered the room. As I took my seat after the hearing teacher pointed to a chair, I noticed that the other children were about my age as the teacher resumed writing on the blackboard. After getting over the shock of a initial new setting, I came to realize what my new teacher was teaching that day.

The teacher had written on the blackboard a list of colors such as gold, gray and silver and a few others. Another list had names of common animals. The lesson for the day was "difficult colors." We were to look at pictures she showed us and write down the appropriate color and name of animal.

Disbelief and confusion reigned in my head. I would have been in the fifth grade had I not been sent here. I knew the names of all the astronauts who have flown in space and today, here I was, being taught new colors I learned years ago.

The transformation was nearly complete. What did I do that was so bad to end up being sent here? I remember thinking I should have tried harder to hear when I was in public school and maybe I would not be here. I was heartbroken as I looked out the second floor window glancing at the tall chain link fencing that ran far as I could see. The thought of running away slipped away when I remembered I lived 200 miles away and felt as if I had done something so bad that my Mom and Dad did not want me anymore. The realization set in, my world had come to an end, and I had nowhere to go.

I was to remain in that 2nd grade class for a few more weeks before I was moved up into the fourth grade. By then the damage had been done. Apparently, the deaf school had the practice of placing a new student in a class with his age group. Perhaps making an adjustment later in the school year instead of evaluation by testing and utilizing placement exams. Nobody bothered to tell me what was going on and I did not feel that it was safe to ask. I already felt enough harm had been dealt me without asking for more.

Perhaps I was a bit spoiled. At the public school my teachers were always asking me if I understood what was going on. I had special speech classes and teachers concerned of my education. I never felt left out or mystified at what was happening to me. But here at this deaf school, I was just another deaf kid. No speech classes anymore. Nobody cared.

My first week on the campus ended up being a lesson of restrictions. Seems like since I first walked, I always rode some sort of a bicycle. It was part of my life and all my friends from the public school went everywhere with them. But, here at this school of 350 students, bikes were banned. The only bikes to be seen were the ones ridden across the street by kids not penalized for being deaf.

Reality continued to set in. I wasn't going anywhere anymore. My whole world was being shrunk into a closely

16

controlled and monitored situation where decisions I once used to make were now being made for me.

Personal radios and television sets were not allowed in the dormitory. There was one small set in the "sitting room" that was usually on something the dorm staff wanted to watch and the volume low not to "disturb" the hearing staff. In the "sitting room" were enough chairs for all the boys on the floor. If the boys were not in their bedrooms, they were expected to be in the "sitting room." Except for school, mealtimes and supervised extra-circular activities, my life was now confined to this area. The only alternative to watching television, (this being before widespread closed-captioning) were a stack of decades-old obsolete magazines donated to the school. Nothing of which a ten-year-old boy would find of interest. By the end of the year I had read them all several times anyway.

Personal items or toys that could not be shared with everybody were rounded up and locked away. I could see that the dorm staff were going to select all my activities outside of school hours and individualism, which was my nature, was not going to be allowed. Outside world contact barely existed. "Warehousing kids" accurately describes the conditions.

My whole life prior to coming to this place, I had never once considered myself "deaf." I always knew that I had a hearing loss and needed to wear a hearing aid, but I took it in stride much the same way other people need to wear glasses. I considered myself the same as everybody else and the term "deaf" never applied to me.

I remember staring at deaf children who were using sign language before being sent to this institution and thinking it was good that I wasn't "deaf."

A CHILD SACRIFICED

But now here I was, dumped together with "them." Confined to the school grounds, segregated from the mainstream world. Forced to learn sign language and live in a dormitory with strangers. Separated from my Mom, Dad, brothers and childhood friends. Placed in demeaning classes. Never being able to do what normal people do. No more bike rides, no more building forts, no more watching space launches. And now I was also "deaf."

I was born with normal hearing. I was about three years old when my hearing started to deteriorate. By age 5, I had a 85 to 95 db hearing loss in both ears. Fortunately, I had already developed language and speech skills before my hearing loss arrested further development.

Before entering pre-school I was fitted with a hearing aid. Although I clearly remember hating it, but eventually ended up wearing it nearly all the time. Being deprived of a sense was not to my liking, so the bulky electronic device was tolerated.

Although my Mom had hearing loss similar to mine, and knew sign language, (along with her parents and numerous other relatives) our family communicated by voice only and I never learned sign language until that first day at the deaf school. My Dad had normal hearing and had one brother who was also hard-of-hearing and two others with normal hearing.

At the public school I attended, I had an hour a day with a speech therapist. Along with extra concern for me by my first and second grade teachers in the public school, the usage of a amplification at an early age, and the usage of voice communication only at home contributed to my having a normal language development in spite of a very severe hearing loss.

A CHILD SACRIFICED

My childhood prior to coming to the deaf school was filled with happiness and fun. The days were full of adventures and challenges. I had future plans and dreams. My hearing disability barely existed. There was not anything I could not do, it seemed. Life was good to me.

My first grade teacher and especially my second grade teacher in the public school had genuine concern for their students. If any of their students were to fail later in life, it certainly was not anything that happened in their early school years. The biggest impact was the introduction of music into my life. The teacher, for the first hour of class every morning would play the piano and sing childhood songs and contemporary hits of the day, stressing an importance on class participation.

By the time I was in the third and fourth grade at the public school, extra-circular activities started to have an impact in the way of social skills and a diversified education. There was Cubs Scouts, roller skating and swimming lessons. At school, band instrument music lessons, papier mache projects, and even though I hated it, square dancing came into play. Once, a select few of us with a strong interest in music, were chosen to learn Christmas songs in order to go caroling at senior citizen centers during the Christmas season. I remember a visitor came to school once for the purpose of teaching us to sing a certain Christmas song in German.

The rest of my times were spent with my neighborhood friends. One of my friends and classmate at school and I, always had numerous construction projects going on. By the time I was in the fourth grade at the public school, we had built a fort in my friend's backyard, one behind the back fence at my house, another up in a tree that our parents did not know too much about and a fourth we started to build with scraps from a subdivision under development. My Dad tore that one down after it started to get taller than all the new houses going up around it.

Other times, we would be on our bikes riding to areas further and further away from our houses. For eight year olds, the sense of discovery and curiosity overwhelmed the danger we might face from our parents for exceeding the boundary of the "immediate neighborhood."

One of our discoveries was Trouble Lake. In deep woods near our neighborhood, only a few kids and supposedly, no parents knew of its existence. Tales of snakes and other water creatures kept most kids away. The trail to the lake resembled the Amazon rain forest to an eight-year-old. Things crawled and slithered along the trail.

We built a raft and went on imaginary expeditions, and when the lake froze over during the winter, we pretended to conquer Alaska. Our creature-fearing friends were left behind.

Once, during a heavy snowstorm, we were checking out the lake and my little brother ended up in water up to his waist. I do not remember the excuse I gave my parents, but it must have been good because I did not have to mention Trouble Lake, named after the trouble you would be in if your parents found out you were there.

On occasion, we would go with my Mom to visit her culturally deaf friends. In once instance, we visited a deaf couple who had a deaf son attending a "special" school for the deaf in another part of the state. Their son came home once every few weeks for the weekend and it would be my first time meeting him.

He did not have any speech ability and I did not know sign language. The hearing aid that was helping me overcome a hearing loss was of no use in this circumstance. I thought how glad I was to not be like him and never once thought I was "deaf" like him.

It was in instances like this that parents of deaf children had seeds sown by members of the deaf culture encouraging them to send their child to a state residential school for the deaf and convincing them it being the best possible option for their deaf child.

This culturally deaf couple were so eager to bring another deaf child whom they did not even know into their culture regardless of the consequences, which if in error, would be difficult to reverse. This is typical of leaders and members of the deaf culture trying to preserve their culture. I had no idea they were conspiring to send me to this deaf school.

During the summer before entering the deaf school in the fall, I was still unaware of the changes that lie in store for me. Part of the summer was spent at my grandparents house across the country. Days were spent building yet more forts, swimming, watching lightning from the evening thunder storms and catching fireflies.

Late at night I'd go down into the basement and listen to the transistor radio my grandpa gave me. I would hold it to my ear and would be fascinated how clear I could hear things and the variety of the medium.

Little did I know a cruel trick was being played on me. In a few weeks that radio would be the only thing I would have left from my childhood and my only connection to the world I would be taken from.

A CHILD SACRIFICED

CHAPTER TWO
THE STATE RESIDENTAL SCHOOL FOR THE DEAF

The teacher I was re-assigned to the first year at the deaf school was by far the poorest teacher I would ever have. She was a hearing woman with only rudimentary skills in sign language. The woman was nearly incapable of understanding her own students. She could not conduct an in-depth discussion on any subject she taught for the benefit of her students.

Typically, she would have us read a textbook while she wrote questions on the board for us to copy after the reading assignment. During the major portion of the class hour, she had only said one word to us, "copy," then pointed at the blackboard. The class seemed to consist of mostly "busy work" to keep us occupied.

She disciplined this class of 13-and 14-year-olds by locking students in dark closets and crudely tapping the students on the head with a yard stick to establish authority and get their attention.

Once, while standing behind the desk of one of her students to check his writing assignment, she was screaming at the student for writing the wrong answer down. Knowing that the student could not hear her, and mistakenly, assuming no one else in the class could either, she yelled obscene language at him referring to his lack of intelligence and his hearing disability.

Another incident occurred when the audio-visual assistant came in, who happened to be a deaf man, to help the teacher with a film projector. The teacher mumbled under her breath that she did not need his help as she greeted him. After the projector was set up properly, she thanked him, but as soon as the deaf man turned to leave the room she yelled at him "that damned man."

I remember the disbelief I felt when I discovered that one of the text book being used in her class was published in 1915. The lesson I learned from that day was to promptly turn to the copyright page of any book I picked up to see how old it was.

Once a week during the school week there was a library visit to check out a book or two. I usually finished reading it the first day and would often borrow my roommates books to read. I ended up learning a lot about presidents and historical leaders, not because I had an interest, but my roommate did. Eventually the school librarian showed an interest in me and let me check out four or five books at a time. Later I was able to stop in the library anytime I wanted to check out the latest books and magazines. The librarian always made me feel welcome and it was the only place at the deaf school that resembled the mainstream world I was taken from.

The second year at the deaf school was somewhat better, but then there was no place to go but up. The instructor, recently hired, was a hearing man and actually was a pretty good teacher, but he was also a minister and a strict disciplinarian. This eventually proved to be his undoing.

While he was able to communicate with the students and showed concern for them, he crossed the fine line of the separation of church and state. His preoccupation with doling out punishment that was unreasonably excessive, apparently precluded his career as a teacher of the deaf.

Although I was too young to know about the U.S. Supreme Court's ban on school prayer, and this teacher was certainly not going to tell us about it, I never had to pray in the public school. Something was not right, but I just played along for a while.

Not to say that some of the disciplinary actions were undeserved for us, but the instructor did not have a grasp of the structured nature of dormitory life. For discipline he would require repetitive written assignments. This was all repetitive work just to consume time away from us on other things. In the dorm, we simply did not have "free" time to do this. Our time at the dorm was structured for us. To find time would meant missing meals, which meant more trouble or doing it in other teachers classes. If it was not completed, it would be "doubled."

Everybody in my class was constantly struggling to find time to complete the work. All my classmates were on the older boy's floor at the dorm which meant I went to bed about an hour earlier than they did and had even less time to do the work. After a few months, I decided I'd had enough.

I simply refused to go to class. During a meeting with some of the school administrators, I told of our experiences. For the rest of the year, there was no more school prayer and repetitive writing assignments. A few years later the teacher left the school for a position better suited for his beliefs.

The deaf school required all the students to take an hour or two of vocational classes each school day. Some were typical and traditional "shop" classes, but it seemed too many of them were vocational classes with narrow employment opportunities. Dry cleaning and leather-working to name a few, were taught by instructors who taught nothing else. These classes were taught for years despite the fact that virtually nobody graduating from the deaf school ever got employment in these fields and have long been obsolete employment opportunities. Apparently, the instructors were hired, guaranteed employment until their retirement. The quality of the education for the students often took a lower priority over the concerns of the staff members.

An art-related vocational class was taught by a professional commercial artist. This was a truly beneficial class with many employment opportunities. Unfortunately, the classes were filled with students with skilled art abilities wanting to have fun while some students with a true interest in wanting to learn the commercial art business were cast aside.

The deaf school also had an complete and up-to-date print shop staffed by good instructors. The print shop turned out excellent printed material and publications for the state and the school. Unfortunately, this was done at the expense of the students. While striving for perfection, the students were mostly limited to the mundane tasks while the instructors did most of the finish work. The school had a monthly magazine and yet the students had no editorial voice over contents, style or the finished product. The students were not given the opportunity to learn this factor of the publishing medium. The school magazine was more of a show-piece for the school to use with parents, the state legislative, and educators to give the image of "success" at the school.

The deaf school overlooked potential employment training opportunities for students that were already available on campus. Many students, after graduation, went into these fields due to the demands of the job market. Vocational training opportunities overlooked were: landscaping and grounds maintenance, shipping/receiving and warehousing, child care, teacher's aides, hospital/nurses aide, bookkeeping, secretarial/filing, to name a few. The school staffed a media center for years with assistants before realizing the learning opportunity for students. I feel its safe to say more former deaf students of this school are employed in the areas overlooked than actually have a job learned from a vocational class they once took.

In junior high, there was a reprieve from the string of "abnormal" experiences. I felt less restricted and more inclined to not dwell much on being here, but rather to get through this deaf school experience.

A highlight of that year, although it may seem insignificant to others, was the science class. While science was my favorite subject and I enjoyed fooling around in the lab, I looked forward to the class mainly because of the stereo system the hearing instructor had in the class. Every day for a whole hour I was able to listen to records he had through a set of headphones. I own several CD's today of records I first heard in that class.

I remembered feeling a kind of loss for the students at the school. Many of them could hear so much better than me, yet had poor hearing discrimination. They would never experience music the way I could. All the childhood songs they never knew, the Christmas carols that made the Christmas experience, and the contemporary music that would be left behind. I later came to realize that this lost culture was insignificant to them, yet would have been devastating to me. It was a rude reckoning. Surely, I did not belong there.

In most cases, it appeared to me the typical new hard-of-hearing student at the deaf school will discontinue use of his hearing aid.

In many cases, the deaf members of the facility will not encourage the use of a hearing aid as they are members of the deaf culture themselves. They have a preference to see the deaf students grow up and become more like them and join their culture.

Very few specialists will dispute with the fact that a child with some hearing ability must use amplication to retain his speech ability, hearing discrimination and language development. The effects would be very difficult to reverse after prolonged discontinuance.

As I mentioned before, there were quite a number of students with better hearing ability than mine, but never learned speech or hearing discrimination. Others simply let their skills deteriorate from a lack of use. This latter group is especially disturbing when the school allows this happen. To once have tools to help survive in the hearing society only to later lose them in the deaf school atmosphere is a tragedy.

An example of this clearly illustrates the point. When I entered the deaf school, two other hard-of-hearing kids about my age entered the same year. Since none of us knew sign language, we talked to each other by voice during the first week of school not to feel so left out. We eventually ended up in different classes and dorms and did not remain close.

A CHILD SACRIFICED

However, by the time I had graduated seven years later, both of them had long since discontinued use of a hearing aid and could only speak in a series of one syllable words and grunts. They could no longer understand speech. We had to communicate in sign language, period. While on the other hand, I wore my hearing aid every awakening moment during the same period and during my Senior year, I remember being able to interpret a college basketball tournament on the radio for some of the students following the games in spite of having the worse hearing for a hard-of-hearing student at the deaf school. This has convinced me the leaders of the deaf culture calling for a lower priority for speech and hearing training, are way off base.

During the first two years at the deaf school, there were no speech classes. I found it to be strange because at the public school, I had a daily speech therapist who constantly reminded me of the importance of continued speech training even though it was at the expense of an hour of regular class time.

At the state deaf school, where one would virtually assume a special department for the continual training and development of speech in hearing-impaired children, it barely existed. Only a few teachers taught any speech classes and this occurred mostly in the upper levels. This was a state school for the **deaf** and they meant it literally. They were not set up to handle hard-of hearing children. Any ability to speak upon arrival here was eventually lost, or simply deteriorated. It would be a challenge for the school to come up with students whose speech had actually improved during the their time on campus. I would note here that expansion of vocabulary does not constitute an improvement.

A CHILD SACRIFICED

There was a full-time audiologist at the school with an assistant. I saw him once a year for 20 minutes. As a prime candidate to benefit from his expertise, it never came.

Whenever I asked about the non-existence of these classes, I would be told that my speech was very good and didn't need it. And I eventually believed it. It wasn't until after I graduated and was exposed to the hearing society, I began to realize that my speech was not quite that good after all. In fact it was quite bad. The years at the deaf school took a toll. My speaking ability was as good as a 4th grade hearing kid. I discovered that a hearing disability is easy to overcome, a speech disability is not. Nowadays, if I am discriminated against by the mainstream hearing society, it is almost always because of my poor speech.

Speech was not a priority item at the deaf school. Commonly used words such as "interpreter," and the name of the large river flowing next to the school was mispronounced by me for years in the deaf school, but was quickly pointed out to me after I graduated. Not once, did any of the hearing teachers care enough to set me straight.

This is not to condemn the few teachers who taught speech at the deaf school. In junior high I had 15 minutes a week on a one-to-one basis, with the instructor being quite good in his efforts, but it was simply not enough time for a person with a hearing disability such as mine.

In high school things improved a bit as I often would get one or two hours a week, but by then the damage had been done and it was an uphill battle to overcome. The instructor in high school was excellent and seemed to be wasting her talent. Upon reaching high school level, most of the students with any hearing ability were "lost causes." There was no hope to even approach normalcy. It is not possible to teach someone speech in high school after years of neglect and expect useful results.

Another problem was that too much of the speech class time was spent trying to learn lip-reading. To this day I can barely lip-read yet most of my communication is done using speech. It is said that to lip-read is an art, it cannot be taught.

While it may have been true of my having the best speech among students at the time, however compared to a group of hearing students, I would have had by far the worse speech. Just because a hard-of-hearing child has "good" speech is no excuse to discontinue or diminish speech training.

I run into many culturally deaf adults today who have a much better hearing ability than mine, yet cannot speak, never learned to speak or simply stopped speaking. While individual responsibility can take some blame, the state residential deaf schools must assume some of the responsibility for this.

Parents of deaf children need to be aware of this ominous reality. If your small child has any hearing ability at all (not being totally or profoundly deaf), placing a child into this type of school is questionable and probably should be avoided at all cost. To do so, your child might as well be totally deaf. Older children should only resort to such a place as a last resort.

The tragic result of a hearing loss early in life is not so much the loss of a sense, but rather, difficulty in obtaining a language. With normal channels for communication closed or obstructed, language development is slowed. The importance of amplication during the speech and language development phase of a child before school age is vital for any hope of approaching normalcy.

31

A CHILD SACRIFICED

If this does not happen due to ignorance on the part of the parents, or the incorrect method selected to educate the child, more often than not, the child will spend the rest of his life trying to master English but never achieving perfection.

Most of the students at a typical residential school for the deaf will graduate with English language skills 4 to 8 years behind their hearing counterparts. While educators do not agree on exact numbers, they seem to range in that area.

A deaf child would be very fortunate to have a master of English approaching the high school level upon graduation from the deaf school. I need not say the importance of this to succeed in our society. English language skills, more than a hearing disability, determines the kind of life one achieves.

This is not to say it was the fault of some of the teachers at the deaf school. At the high school level, the most devoted and dedicated teacher was our English teacher. Totally deaf himself, he had the difficult task of educating these deaf youngsters into mastering a language in order to cope in the mainstream world, yet knowing at best, he could only marginally succeed. Perhaps, by being deaf himself and by the example he set, dedicatedly pushing for effort, he was able to motivate harder work from the students than any one else. There was no slacking off in his class because he left no doubt in our minds that knowledge of this stuff was seriously important and necessary. Years after our graduation, most of my classmates still had admiration for him and his genuine concern for our futures.

This deaf school primarily seemed to favor the method of educating the students using ASL. (American Sign Language) Although the official method was "Total Communication," (a combination of sign language utilizing the signing of each word and speaking the words at the same time) outside the classroom in the dorm, social functions and extra-circular activities, ASL prevailed.

ASL evolved from first being used by the largely uneducated deaf adults of a century ago into the primary language used and favored by the culturally deaf today. Basically, it is English broken down into its simplistic form. It is mostly graphic in form and is easily learned, especially for the uneducated or without language formation.

For example, to sign "house," one makes a shape of a house with his hands. To make a phrase in ASL, one would sign "me go store," when one meant "I am going to the store" in English. Another example would be to sign "eat finish," to mean "I already ate." ASL has is own idioms and although somewhat fluid, rules. One is able to express all their thoughts unrestricted. *not easy consensus for deaf.*

Unfortunately, I believe the simplicity of ASL is self-defeating. Often, a deaf person becomes a master at ASL at the expense of learning English. ASL is their primary language too often and English becomes their second language. They would experience English the same way a normal hearing person would learn a second language, such as a difficult language like German or Japanese. One could become quite skilled if effort is there, but never quite mastering it as well as his first language. Also, being fluent in ASL makes it difficult to motivate school age deaf children into mastering another language. Further, there is the problem of some students not actually learning the word the sign represents. Not even mentioned is the difficulty English is to learn as a second language.

The deaf culture argues ASL is a language onto itself and it is all that is needed for a deaf person to be fulfilling in life. However, English is the language one has to learn to be a contributor to our society. It is unreasonable for the deaf culture to expect everyone to learn sign language.

In the intermediate school, there was a popular deaf teacher who had an innovative way to develop the minds of deaf children. With one of the benefits from ASL being a heightened graphics awareness, the instructor took advantage of it to further the education of his students.

Deaf children are predisposed to be attracted to graphics, pictures and illustrations as opposed to the written word. By cutting out pictures from periodicals and posting them on his classroom door and updating them daily, the teacher managed to expose them to the outside world in a way that might have not of otherwise occurred.

Teachers with this kind of concern, unfortunately were exceptions to the rule.

The school for the deaf is operated as a division under the state department of institutions. Prisons and mental hospitals presented the bulk of this state agency. While one could make a case that these are just labels and all state financing comes from the same source, the people running the department of institutions were usually incarceration experts. With the deaf school being a small part of their responsibilities, the priority of the deaf school is diminished.

Many residential schools for the deaf in other states are run under that state's department of education, where there is more focus on education than on warehousing, and there is a higher degree of accountability for the success of the school.

Another factor with being under the department of institutions, was the ease of the agency to transfer mentally retarded deaf children to the school from the state mental hospitals. Sometimes the number of these transfers often presented a rather large ratio, and many students were cheated out of a quality education when some of the school's resources went to baby-sitting these severely retarded transfers. It also makes one think when the powers that be can easily classify a hearing loss and mental retardation in the same category.

Ironically, the director of the state department of institutions once decided to close the deaf school as a cost-cutting measure. The position it being the responsibility of each individual student's home school district to educate them rather than dumping the deaf children on the state.

This did not happen. The culturally deaf community faced with a threat to their culture and staff members concerned for their jobs raised such an uproar that succeeded in circumventing the proposal. The actual concern of the deaf child's education did not come into play much.

Another uproar erupted over the selection of a new superintendent. It was fueled by the deaf community in a rage over the decision by the state to select a long-time employee of the school and well-qualified successor to the post. The deaf community wanted a deaf person. The appointee, the most qualified of the applicants, was hearing.

The job of the superintendent is mostly political, dealing with the state capitol to keep state funding intact. The appointee had been the assistant superintendent for a number of years and actually was the school's point man in the state capitol.

However, heavy-arm tactics of the deaf community prevailed and the position was to be reopened for another selection. The newly appointed superintendent was relieved after a few months and the old one called out of retirement for another year of service during the upheaval.

This incident, which echoes that of the Gallaudet University revolt of a few years back, underlines the point of a lack of understanding by the culturally deaf of the political system. It seems to me deaf children need to be taught that they cannot be making demands at every dislike, but need to work the political system like everybody else. Let the elected officials know your positions and elect politicians that favor your beliefs. Those who renege or lose your trust can be run out of office.

Although it is accredited now, the deaf school was not accredited to meet any standards that would be expected of comparable educational facilities. This presented a problem for a student wanting to enter some colleges. Although Gallaudet University will routinely accept deaf students who pass their exams, the last thing a deaf graduate needs is another closed door because his school did not have credentials.

In high school, I was fortunate to have a deaf teacher having a highly influential effect on me. It was rather subtle and almost subconscious. By the manner in which he talked, I began to become aware that it was acceptable to "challenge authority." Wanting to change what I did not like was permissible in our society and the status quo did not necessarily have to be maintained.

Slowly, I started moving from the camp of the followers and meek into the progressive camp of the outspoken activists. Although the transformation was not complete until after I graduated from the deaf school, it started one day in his class.

A CHILD SACRIFICED

notri ghT?

While perhaps not the right time and place, the instructor would often get into heated debates with the vice-principal over school policy right in the classroom for us to witness. I learned more then about authority and politics right then than I would have ever learned out of a text book.

Many of the students did not quite understand him and felt there was too much criticism. They completely overlooked the opportunity to have more control of their lives.

This is typical of the deaf culture, the resistance to change. The culture is often hostile to anybody attempting to "rock the boat."

A hearing teacher, dedicated to teaching the deaf, talented far beyond the deaf high school level, taught a course that was difficult for the deaf to learn. The double whammy of deaf students trying to understand the text book already having language difficulty, and the concept of the subject the text is explaining, is a big enough hindrance. However, when compounded with the instructors struggling sign language reading skills, the classroom atmosphere often ranged from desperation to heated disputes over communication breakdowns occurring almost daily.

I have often witnessed either the student or the instructor out of desperation, nod to the other they understood, but actually did not, in order to get off that topic. The student is not served when he deliberately choose to not understand the subject after a communication breakdown with the instructor. Eventually the instructor became skilled in his sign language reading ability, but only after the expense of frustrated students for his first few years,

A CHILD SACRIFICED

One long time instructor, another graduate of Gallaudet University, presented a difficult situation for me. He was extremely popular with the students. It was difficult not to enjoy having a conversation with him, but at the same time he was a very poor teacher.

He had no business teaching at the high school level, if at all. Although should be commended for being able to achieve this much in life, having gone to Gallaudet University and later, into this tenured position. But in retrospect, his presence in the school was a disservice to the students.

Fortunately for him, the subject he taught was straightforward, easily understood by deaf students. While it was simple enough to teach, he could not apply what he taught to be used in a situation in real life.

To ensure the success of his students, he would often discretely provide answer-sheets for future upcoming exams given by off-campus concerns. A few students may or may not owe their success in life (at perhaps, the expense of another more deserving person) to unethical behavior on the part of this instructor.

This instructor was the most popular teacher in high school. The class felt more like social hour and we looked forward to it. He was able to make the students feel that he was like one of us. Nobody was about to pass judgment on the quality of education we were receiving while having such a good time. He maintained full social contacts with many of the recent school alumni, and unfortunately, rumors of wild parties, marijuana and alcohol use filtered down to the high school level.

The reason I present all this is because the instructor began to typify to the deaf students what constitutes a leader of the deaf. A popular term used by the students for him was

A CHILD SACRIFICED

"open minded." This was a term that was incorrectly used. Advocating, although subtly, the use of drugs, unethical behavior, and lowered expectations, established for the deaf students the "normalcy" of this type of behavior.

I feel the widespread implications of this cannot be ignored. This impact stays with the student throughout his adult life and explains a lot of the present state of mind and attitudes of many culturally deaf adults. This kind of harm overwhelms any overlooking of this otherwise well liked instructor.

Ironically, and by contrast, there were other deaf instructors who followed the same path through life, educated at Gallaudet, then in a teaching position at the school. One, a former student body government official in college, having complete knowledge of his courses, fully prepared to discuss and apply to real life, was the perfect role model for the deaf students. However, along with some of the other deaf instructors, he was not given the role because they did not meet the student's criteria for being "open minded."

Prior to entering the deaf school, I had a strong interest in astronomy. My dream was to be an astronaut; if precluded because of my deafness, at least I would be an astronomer. I used to read everything I could about astronomy and rockets. My Dad would wake me up in the wee hours of the morning to watch the space launches.

After entering the deaf school, the lack of motivation and information resulted in my losing interest in the subject. By the end of the first year at the deaf school, I was keenly aware of my setback and the dream faded and replaced with the more urgent need of having to survive this deaf school experience.

A CHILD SACRIFICED

Ironically, the school had a college-level sized telescope in storage. When I became aware of its existence in high school, there was nothing I could do to convince anyone to put it to use. The school administration did not want to trust it to a student; the dorm staff did not want to assume responsibility for it. Since the telescope was of no use to anyone during school hours, (with it being daylight and all) it stayed packed in a box in deep storage. More than seven years went by for me at the school and I never saw the thing. Imagine the better course of life some students could have taken, and in my case, perhaps the chance to be less cynical about this school experience, if the opportunity was not blown by the school administration.

The school had a higher priority for staff conveniences and a preference the students develop an interest in dry cleaning and leather-working than trying to reach for the stars.

Seemingly, my only connection to the outside world was my constant listening to my radio. Using a pair of headphones and two twenty-foot extension cords, I had it on all the time. I listened to my favorite station. Knew all the songs, all the disc-jockeys names; I would always hope some listener would call in and request a good song.

I listened for years to events and activities and other on-goings in the major metropolitan area close to the deaf school, yet never actually being there to experience it. There were advertisements of places of businesses, recreational promotions, and sporting events that I heard of for years. Also were changes in the society, political climate changes, headlining topics of the day during newscast, and even traffic reports on freeways.

Imagine how it struck me, many years later, to finally see all the places I heard about for years and knew about so

A CHILD SACRIFICED

Imagine how it struck me, many years later, to finally see all the places I heard about for years and knew about so well. It was a kind of deja vu. It brought the isolation and segregation from the mainstream society into clear focus.

I was fortunate during high school that many of my teachers allowed me to read other books, some not related to the class I was in, during class discussion. Since most of any class discussion at the deaf school consisted of explaining to the student what was not understood during the previous night's reading homework assignment, the teacher often overlooked my not paying attention. This being because I was always ahead of everybody else and had already read the textbook cover-to-cover.

I would often sneak a smaller and different book into the pages of the textbook when asked to pay attention by some teachers and I would usually be left alone after that.

One deaf instructor that I had every morning for all four years in high school, let me read a volume from an encyclopedia every time I got disinterested in the class lecture or discussion. Seems like never once did he ask me to pay attention as he probably assumed I would get a lot more out of my own personal choice in reading material than anything that could transpire in the classroom. By the time I had graduated, I had read every single volume in that encyclopedia several times.

I do appreciate some of the special allowances given to me by some of the instructors, and some of the "accelerated" classes offered to me, that were not usual circumstances. By not having to endure the normal path a deaf child follows in a structure such as the residential school for the deaf, I apparently escaped the shortcomings many of the graduates of this type of school tend to have, so my education did not become a total loss.

Early in my Senior year, I made up my mind that I was not going to Gallaudet University. The college was established for the deaf in Washington D.C. more than a century ago. It is in essence, the continuation of this deaf school life. This time I had control of my fate and I intended to reverse the educational direction that was made for me. I was also aware that I would be making the ultimate insult to the deaf community. Failure of the deaf school experience to convert me to the deaf culture's way of life.

Gallaudet University is revered by the deaf community as the center of the deaf culture. Worthy enough to be accepted at Galluadet is often the high point of a deaf person's life. To have attended Gallaudet (but, not necessarily to have graduated from) places a deaf individual in an elite social class in the deaf culture. For a deaf student to not want any part of this significant institution of the deaf culture is not easily accepted and is often deemed offensive.

At the residential deaf school, all Seniors, with average or better intelligence, are expected to take the exam which is given once a year. The number of students passing the exam from the school and going on to Gallaudet is a source of pride (albeit misplaced) for the staff and administration of the school. A student not going to Gallaudet even though he was accepted, is often considered a "failure" by the deaf facility.

Most of the deaf teachers were alumni of Gallaudet as well as residential deaf schools. In fact, an ominously high number of staff members graduated from this very school which brings up the question of the diversity of my education. The strength in numbers underlines the influence the staff

42

members flex in maintaining the status quo on behalf of the deaf culture.

The day of the Gallaudet exams arrived. Nobody had asked me if I wanted to take the exams, yet all the forms were filled out on my behalf and recommendations were made by the school administrators to complement my test exams. This was to ensure my being accepted by the college. All this in spite of the fact I had mentioned on numerous occasions that I was not going to Gallaudet.

The ten students taking the exams headed out to the door to the conference room where the exams were being held. I stayed in my chair and told my homeroom teacher I was not going to take the exams. He said that it was my choice and had a look on his face that told of interesting events about to occur.

Only minutes later, the exam specialist came down to talk me into taking the exam. Shortly there after, she was joined by reinforcements, a few other teachers, (and Gallaudet alumni I might add) which she called in, one by one, in an attempt to convince me. Unable to do so, they all left.

The next thing I knew, the vice-principal was standing in front of me and was mad as hell. After rambling on and on about all her effort and time she put in for me on this, she demanded that I go upstairs and take the exam. I replied saying nobody had asked me if I wanted to take the exam and there was no way I was going to another deaf school. At that point, she turned around and faced the homeroom teacher. She said nothing but the anger in her face spoke volumes. And the exams were given without my presence.

Of course, I was subject to ridicule by many of the deaf teachers in the days following the exam, as well as some of the dorm staff members. This also reached beyond the confines of the campus. They would taunt me and reply that I was afraid I would not pass the exam, or that I was "chicken," etc. I came to believe they did it with intent of malice as only weeks ago I scored the highest grade in the whole school on the Stanford Achievement Tests and my grade point average for that year was a perfect score. Little did these people know that they had sowed seeds of anger that would eventually grow into this book, returning to haunt them for their past misdeeds.

Again, as I was to find out much later, the deaf culture does not take a liking to someone who wants to "rock the boat." The resistance to change is very strong in the deaf community and the fact I seriously did not want to go to Gallaudet was a rejection of their way of life and was unacceptable to them. The deaf employees at the school felt it was justifiable to seriously ridicule a 16-year-old student in retaliation.

I can recall only the homeroom teacher assured me it was okay if I did not want to go to Gallaudet and go elsewhere. Others mentioned I should have just taken the exam, got accepted, then go ahead and enter another college and would have avoided the wrath of the deaf community. Apparently, I preferred the confrontation than to play along with their little game.

Incidentally, we found out two months later only two students passed the exams that year. This was embarrassing to the staff and a dark day in history for this deaf school. While I had no intent to not take the college exams out of revenge, but somehow, I would not be telling the truth if I said I felt no pleasure upon hearing the news. By that time, the deaf community had exposed itself to me in full circle and pieces started to fall together of a *community scrambling to preserve itself and I was being used to achieve that agenda.*

CHAPTER THREE
Broken Family Bond

The residential dormitory at the school for the deaf presents the most influence the deaf culture has to mold a child into their image. Having been the by-product of deaf residential schools for centuries, the deaf culture need not do much other than to ensure such residential schools continue to exist. The segregated nature of the dormitory life will take care of the rest.

While there may be a place for schools dedicated to teaching the deaf in our society, I feel placing a child in a *residential* school for the deaf is not in the best interest of a deaf child. The leaders of the deaf culture would have you believe otherwise.

The main concern of parents of deaf children is focused on the education the child receives, and not much concern is given to the "dorm life;" subsequentially, the deaf culture the child absorbs.

The child is separated from his family and the, perhaps already fragile, family bond is severely broken. The child will bond with the other deaf children and they will become the child's new family. The dorm staff members becomes the primary influence on the child's life and the parents take a back seat. And quite often, these staff members will be culturally bad situation.

deaf themselves and the child has no option, but to absorb the culturally deaf way of life for better or worse.

The influence of the dorm staff members cannot be diminished. While the better paying positions at the school in the educational department attracts higher caliber personnel, (at least in theory) the staff at the dormitories and their meager pay scales leaves a lot to be desired.

While some dorm staff members were dedicated to deaf children, many were there just for the paycheck and the deaf children were seemingly just in the way.

Many were under-educated and ignorant. Concern for the deaf child had a low priority. Communication was the biggest shortcoming. Many did not sign. Others that could, often were not able to understand the deaf child's signs. All too often, a group of children would be punished because the dorm staff member could not understand them and discover who actually caused the problem.

The dorm staff members own personal bias were extended to the children. African-Americans were called "niggers" and "colored." Hispanics were described as "dirty" and "low class." Members of the Jewish faith were pointed out as "greedy," and "troublemakers." Even other deaf people, educated in the "oral" method, were accused of having made a bad choice in life and were looked down upon.

Disciplinary actions, for a long time, especially for the younger students, were whippings. Kids being disciplined often lined up with their pants removed for their whippings at a set time of the day set aside for this. Overzealous staff members sometimes used their own belts, being more lethal, instead of the "official" paddle. Others often whipped several innocent children to ensure the person who actually caused the trouble got spanked when there was a doubt of which child was actually guilty. Other crude methods to discipline the children were to have them kneel in the hall, often on broomsticks, for long stretches of time.

To this day, I feel as if I had once been in prison, having been a witness to these type of punishments that was being dealt to the deaf children during my early years at the school.

Some dorm staff members were cruel and crude with the children. In one incident, a 13 year-old boy was caught by a non-dorm staff member experimenting with homosexual behavior. Instead of the facility providing counseling to help him understand his sexuality, a relief dorm staff member took it upon himself to "rectify" a situation by exhibiting his own personal bias during a special dorm meeting called for the purpose of embarrassing the student.

The deaf staff member told all the boys how his family and the boy's family were close friends and told of having spent the summer together doing activities. And now, he was embarrassed his family was involved with that boy who was a "homo." He told the boy his own family is now ashamed of him. And finally, he told all the boys on the floor, they too, should be ashamed if they were friends with him.

The precedent established that day for the boys was the acceptability of hate. The staff member instilled his own narrow-mindedness and bigotry into the minds of these youngsters with a vivid and memorable presentation.

Late at night, there were night-watchpersons, usually hearing and knew no sign language. They would often arbitrarily punish everyone in a room or on a ward, as a solution to a communication gap. One watchperson, yelled foul language at the children habitually, assuming that the deaf children were not hearing him. It was from this man, I learned my first four-letter-words and got a daily dose of the ugly side of adults.

Often, the dorm staff will subject the students to their own misguided sense of justice. This gives the students the impression of acceptable behavior and the deaf child often carries it into adult life.

In one case, the dorm director punished all the boys in the dormitory based on circumstantial evidence for a crime that may actually have been caused by someone outside the dorm.

Apparently, tires of the personal vehicle of a relief dorm staff member were slashed while he was on duty in our dorm. Nobody came forward to admit the crime during a dorm meeting called for that reason.

The dorm director overlooked the fact the houseparent mostly worked the older boy's dorm and parked his vehicle in the same place every day by our dorm. Also, the older boys were more likely to do this kind of retaliating towards a staff member. Also ignored, was the opportunity that it was caused by someone off campus as the dorm was next to a public housing project, somewhat rundown, and home to many hearing juvenile delinquents.

With his sense of justice, the dorm director took all the money the students earned from activities all year, earmarked for a special end-of-year field trip, and bought a new set of tires for the crime victim.

Time and time again, I see these kinds of miscarriages of justice in the adult deaf culture and they are deemed perfectly normal. The roots of these misguided concepts often began during dormitory life.

A hearing dorm staff member for the grade-school-aged boys presented a concern for me and another student. Although we were only about 12 years old, we could clearly see she was using too much force in handling kids under her supervision. Perhaps it was not too apparent to her superiors.

She was in her 60's with only rudimentary sign language skills and having no ability to understand it. Her method of supervision consisted of mostly slapping the kids and prodding them with a ruler, much like the way one would use a cattle prod. She also screamed at them in foul language, especially when her co-workers were not around.

It came to a point where we approached the dorm director. The director brushed us off by saying she has devoted her whole life to the deaf and we were told to be "understanding."

Perhaps she was reprimanded, to give the dorm director the benefit of the doubt, but we were left with the impression that "officially," her behavior was acceptable to the school. However, thankfully for my having a basis for comparison, I believed otherwise. Nevertheless, she continued in her ways for a few more years until her death finally spared deaf children the cattle prod.

This type of abuse was apparently widespread. A few years after I graduated, several staff members were asked to retire for physically abusing the children and the director of the primary boys dorm was dismissed. There have also been firings at other state residential deaf schools involving both physical and sexual abuse and a case can be made for residential schools not being exempt from the undesirable elements in our society. Parents are often unaware of staff-level on-goings.

Selection of some of the social functions arranged for the students can also be questioned. One such occurrence was a religious event held on the school campus by an off-campus concern. It was open to the general public and the students were invited to participate.

As it turned out, it was some kind of sermon and rally presented by some "faith healers." An interpreter provided a sign language account of the proceedings for the deaf students. Halfway through the event, several people were called to the stage having "disabilities." First a "blind" person was made to see again, then a person in a wheelchair was able to walk again.

At this point, the "minister" had the whole audience in a captured spell and then pointed out a deaf child to come to the stage. This person was a friend of mine and I knew he was totally deaf and could not speak.

Now, with the eyes of the whole audience watching, and with a convincing performance by the minister doing faith healing rituals, he nodded his head when prompted by the minister asking if he could now hear. The whole audience broke into applause and cheers having seen someone "cured."

Immediately, one of the deaf staff members, perhaps the wisest of all the adults present, stood up and ordered all the deaf students to leave. He said the "cartoon" we were witnessing was not appropriate for the students.

It was incredible the school allowed this event to take place on the campus of a publicly funded educational facility and in the presence of the students. The moral integrity of the school was saved by a "lowly" relief dorm staff member.

A CHILD SACRIFICED

There was also a problem of hazing among the older students. To keep the knowledge from reaching the staff members and parents, pain was often inflicted in a way that the victim would be too embarrassed to talk to staff members about it, let alone parents. There was also the threat of further hazing from the students.

I witnessed one student suffer from embarrassment and discomfort, over and over, until there was a painful injury before seeking relief from his parents. The lower the student's intelligence, the more likely it would occur. Mentally retarded transferees were the biggest targets.

These mentally retarded transferees were also victims of sexual abuses by some of the students. Sometimes, they would be abused by someone for their own gratification or for the amusement of an audience. This often accounts for the "first lesson" in sex education the students are exposed to.

Often a degree of fear was instilled in some of the children who were otherwise perfectly innocent. An example of this, once, late at night, in the older boys dorm, someone made a mess of the dorm staff office. Among other things, flashlights were turned on and the telephones were hidden. Since this mischief had the signature of someone I knew, he confirmed it when I asked him. He had a beef with the dorm staff over a personal issue.

The next morning, there was an uproar over the dead batteries and the inconvenience of missing phones. Later, there was yet another dorm meeting, called by the director to try to weed out the troublemaker.

With his very inquisitive style of interrogating, he was able to get two boys to admit to causing the trouble, neither of which actually had anything to do with it other than the proximity of their bedrooms to the office. It was just incredible, knowing there was someone else chuckling at the meeting also. The deaf dorm director's heavy-handed management style moved the innocent to plead guilty for a better fate than the one they feared if they continued to plead innocent.

This is truly sad social commentary as one student, who was present at this meeting, later in life pleaded guilty to a felony he did not commit as part of a plea bargain that would gain his immediate release from jail. It took lawyers years to convince the courts this innocent person pleaded guilty out of a false fear acquired during his early years at a residential school for the deaf.

At this residential school for the deaf, the older the student, the more privileges extended to the student. By high school level, there were off-campus passes and increased socializations with female students. Prior to high school, the boys and girls are for the most part, segregated.

The students at the deaf school were denied the American teenager's love affair with automobiles. Rules to ban them on campus, along with many other such policies were made seemingly for the convenience of the staff than for any concern or benefit for the students.

An example of this, the hearing dorm staff constantly turned down the television sets watched by the students, saying it was "too loud." Forgotten was this was a **deaf** school and the students were **deaf**! Instead of using ear plugs, it was easier to cut off the culture and experience of sound for the students.

This was especially a problem with stereos. Even the profoundly deaf can appreciate some form of music through vibration from the speakers. But nearly every confrontation with the staff members ended with the plug being pulled. I would just go back to using headphones to please the dorm staff. Bringing the issue up with the dorm director would bring the standard response of "a bad impression for visitors" or some other public relations excuse.

It nearly goes without saying, the younger the child, the less privileges they had, compared to their hearing counterparts, and the more likely they were to be treated like cattle. To observe the dorm staff members in the primary children's dorms, they always seemed to be rounding them up and herding them out from one place to another.

There were no deaf staff members in the primary boy's dorm and few knew sign language well. While I was fortunate to never have actually lived in the primary dorm, I have heard enough from those who have and from what I have been able to observe from across campus with my own eyes, I have reached this conclusion: concerned parents should take note, if the deaf school is your last option for your child, the older the better.

If I had started my early schooling at the deaf school, I seriously doubt that I would have the same success I enjoy today. By not having the basis for comparison, I would probably be more favorable towards the deaf culture. It would be difficult then to criticize the only way of life I would have only known, even if faulty. The outside hearing world would have seemed so distanced and unobtainable with my having never lived in it. This book would never have been written.

basic knowledge
of sign l.
only needed

A CHILD SACRIFICED

CHAPTER FOUR
SURVIVAL

In order to survive the segregated deaf school environment, I engaged in various forms of mischief. In doing so, I would be pre-occupying myself and momentarily forgetting where I was. I never did anything morally wrong, but rather, did things that caused disruptions or inconveniences for the staff members. As I found out later, other students of the school had done the same for the identical reasons. These momentary escapades preserved my sanity. I found great amusement in observing perplexed staff members.

Telephones were my favorite pastimes. I found a way to record ordinary TDD (telephone device for the deaf) conversations on my cassette player. I also devised a way to play back pre-recorded conversations over the TDD machines. This only worked with the deaf staff members as the hearing staff would hear the recording being blasted through the wall from my stereo system. They were often quite perplexed to receive a phone call with an exact text to a call they made earlier in the week.

This adventure came to an end when a dorm director became suspicious, and came to me and said he had no idea what was happening, but I was the only one clever enough to do such things.

The dorm staff never found out the source of a siren, seemingly coming on and off at random in spurts. Hidden in a crawl space several floors above the phone line it was tied into, it sounded when a certain phone was ringing. Since it was answered rather immediately by supervisory personnel several floors below, the dorm staff members never made the connection between the phone, the siren, and the automatic silence.

One day in the older boy's dorm, we got a new dorm staff member. We did not know anything about him other than he was very fluent in ASL. Usually a hearing person is not capable of being fluent enough in sign language to pass for a deaf person. However, this one signed so well. We had no idea if he was actually hearing or deaf.

I decided to put him through a hearing test to find out. There were two phones in the office, so I called from one phone and dialed the number of the other. Immediately after the first ring he got up to answer the phone. I then quietly hung up. Everybody in the room now smiled having known of my plan. He returned to his chair unaware the deaf people in the room had made him the subject of a little test.

Interesting I thought, usually people take advantage of the deaf not being able to hear, but this time, the deaf took advantage of a hearing person being able to hear. This dorm staff member had obtained his sign language skills from his deaf parents.

A CHILD SACRIFICED

Once, a couple of my friends were walking back from a store near the campus and we were engaged in discussion of the fine points of hitchhiking. While it wasn't permitted, my friend offered to find us a ride on a dare he had a "natural" ability to hitch rides.

He walked out to the curb, snapped his fingers and stuck his thumb out. Sure enough, a car pulled over and stopped right in front of us almost immediately. My friend opened the back door for me and got in the front passenger side himself. I was about 14 years old and was certainly impressed with hitchhiking already.

However, I knew something wasn't right once in the car. The driver was an elderly lady with fear in her eyes and shaking visibly as she watched "home sign language" used by my friend to describe where we wanted to go. On the way to the campus, we wondered why she stopped to give three long haired teenagers a ride if she was going to be this afraid?

Once we reached our designation, we thanked the lady and waved goodbye. Looking relieved, she turned the car around and headed back to the direction we had come from. Then it dawned on us that we had been standing in front of her house when we were hitchhiking and the elderly lady had just simply pulled over to park in front of her house. We unintendedly forced our way into her car and made her take us somewhere.

One pretty amusing time in high school occurred in Literature class. The instructor had the class view several short films then assigned us to pick a film and write about it.

One of the films had a lively musical soundtrack with several rock songs on it, and along with another hard-of-hearing classmate, I picked that one in order to view it again several times with the true purpose of listening to the music. Since the instructor was totally deaf, he was unaware of the soundtrack, and of course, our primary reason of wanting to watch it each day. Even after the first viewing of the day, we would rewind it and play it again with the projector lamp off just to listen to it over and over.

By the end of the week, the instructor was impressed with the amount of time we were devoting to his assignment. However, our game came to an abrupt end when one of the hearing teachers came in the classroom saying he had been hearing that same music all week and wondered where it was coming from. Boy, was our faces red when our instructor looked at us and the movie projector we had hidden partially behind a door, running with the projector lamp off!

Due to my young age, I didn't play on most varsity sport teams at the deaf school until I was a Senior. However, I was able to be a part of the activities by being an official scorer or statistician for the team or covering the sport sometimes in the capacity as sports writer for the school monthly magazine.

At times, I often wondered if my presence on the team was for the purpose of providing a fourth player for games of pinochle played on the bus rides to the away games. The coach and assistant coach along with two students, had a tradition of playing on the trips to the games for years until one graduated. My position on the basketball team became starting pinochle player.

After a few years of playing pinochle, I actually became pretty good as the coaches cheated by whispering and the other student and I devised ways to overcome that.

A CHILD SACRIFICED

I did get a varsity letter at the end of the year, but probably should have gotten a "deck of cards" pin to put on my varsity jacket. *included yes.*

Having an interest in astronomy, I knew of ways in and out of the dormitory in the middle of the night in order to get out and make observations and perhaps take a walk down to the lake without getting detected. While only 13 years old and already a night owl, I knew of the night watchmen and security people's schedules well enough that I was able to see the astronomical events like meteor showers, comets and eclipses in spite of a 9 o'clock bedtime. I would stuff clothing in my bed and be on my way.

All that came to an end when I went out one night with two friends. Our adventure took an ugly turn when we attempted to return to the dorm. Back inside, we realized one of us couldn't climb back up the steel filigree leading to the top of the terrace. Not wanting to leave him behind to the wrath of the dorm director, we went to the rescue of our friend.

Unbeknownst to us, the night watchman heard my friend make a racket trying to get up to the second floor and stood out of sight waiting to see if there were any accomplices. Not knowing he was listening for us, we played right into his hands as we climbed down from the terraces attempting a rescue. In a way, we were taken advantage of due to our hearing loss, but it was a good lesson in life to know and learn to compensate for it in the future. *no u went wrong.*

In high school once, the junior class had a novel idea for raising money. They went to people's houses and asked if they wanted their cars washed and the class would do it hoping for donations. The class advisor, making an ill-advised

59

decision, picked the person in the class with the best "speaking ability" to solicit people wanting cars washed while the rest of the class did the actual washing of the cars.

The guy with the best speaking ability actually was pretty bad. He could only speak broken rudimentary English and left out key words sometimes. In some cases, he actually said to people answering the door of their homes, "do you want your car?" leaving out the vital key word "washed." Naturally they would respond with "yes." He took it to mean they wanted their car washed.

As you can guess, a few cars got washed without real permission before the class adviser caught on to what was happening.

Sometimes, a few of us would go hangout at a street corner late at night near the campus, waiting for a police car to cruise by. When one would eventually appear, we would all then scatter and make a run for it. More often than not, the patrol car would follow us on campus, driving over the curb and onto the grounds with lights flashing and sirens wailing. We were running for our lives, half expecting to be hit by bullets. Knowing the shortcuts on campus, we made it to our dormitory undetected.

I remember looking out the dorm window with a dorm staff member, trying to act as dumbfounded as he was about why the city police would be conducting a ground search of our campus.

Along with a classmate, we hid various speakers we "confiscated" from sources around campus and hid them in radiators on several floors of the dorm. We secretly wired them to a stereo system and at night we would manipulate the system to turn music on then off again when the dorm staff members turned on the lights on the floors, looking for the source of blasting rock music. The dorm staff members were completely befuddled while the boys in the dorm were unaware of what was transpiring.

During a cold spell with the temperature in the single digits, the whole student body was warned of not going down to the lake. Even though it was frozen over, the school did not want to assume the responsibility. Yet somehow, the lure of the ice attracted about a group of twenty of us to get up in the middle of the night, bundle up, sneak out of the dorm in single file, like soldiers on a mission, down the hill towards the lake. With a 35 miles-per-hour Arctic blast across the lake in our face and the near full moon above, we reached our objective. After sacrificing a member to test the ice thickness, we soon were experiencing the forbidden ourselves.

Such escapades made the deaf school experience more bearable and time pass quicker. Not occurring too soon, my time at the deaf school had come to an end. After graduation, I entered a local community college in my home town which was also a branch of the large state university located upstate. I choose it because of my determination to show I was perfectly able to function at a mainstream hearing educational facility. I guess I also wanted to show that it was a mistake to send me to the deaf school in the first place.

There were no other deaf students there and very few support services for deaf students. I picked an adviser who had no experience with "disabled" students. I wanted to be treated like everybody else on campus and I got what I wanted.

A CHILD SACRIFICED

By utilizing a notetaker so I could concentrate on the lectures, I found that I picked right up where I left off in the 4th grade. For the first time in seven years I was listening to instructors in a class room lecturing by voice only. It was just as I remembered it. Some were funny, others were boring and most of the instructors cared about the success I had with their classes, unlike what I was lead to believe about hearing colleges from some of the teachers at the deaf school. I passed every class I completed that year. By the end of the school year most, but not all, of my frustration toward the deaf school had come to pass.

This is not to say that others could succeed in a totally hearing environment, but it my case, it goes to say the decisions which resulted in my being accepted and placed into the deaf school was a huge mistake in judgment by all the parties involved.

Today, I find myself in the fringe area of the deaf culture. I seem to have found some middle ground between both the deaf culture and the mainstream hearing world. However, I am also accused of being too close to the hearing world for the deaf culture's comfort.

It is difficult for many to live at the fringe area with the pressure from the deaf culture to either commit totally, or go away completely. This is why it is so easy to revert back to the ways of the culturally deaf. With the social attractions of the deaf world, most culturally deaf people, even though sometimes they would like to, won't dare venture out to the fringe of the culture. Since the hearing world isn't about to greet them with open arms, the lure of the deaf culture prevails.

A CHILD SACRIFICED

It takes a strong minded person to make it in both worlds, but sometimes it helps when you feel you don't belong to either one. The plight of the large hard-of-hearing (but not culturally deaf) community is a another book in itself. Outnumbering the culturally deaf by a large margin, these people are not visible to other hard-of-hearing people in our society, thus they aren't able to organize in the same way as the culturally deaf. (The easily visible "calling card" of sign language identifies the culturally deaf to each other.)

Pessimists would describe my world as "no man's land," while optimists would remind me of having the "best of both worlds."

A CHILD SACRIFICED

CHAPTER FIVE
ROOM FOR IMPROVEMENT

In the deaf community today, there is an unwritten rule against publicly criticizing the deaf community. This seems to be due to the fact there is no appealing alternative lifestyle to turn to. The shortcomings of the deaf community are much preferred to than living within the mainstream hearing society. An even worse alternative it seems, is the "oral method" lifestyle, which the deaf culture despises. With no place else to go, members of the deaf community are not likely to cause any kind of "trouble" that might alienate the leaders of the deaf community.

It is common today for many young adult culturally deaf males not even be aware of their behavior towards females, (especially verbally) which would be construed as sexual harassment in the mainstream hearing society. It is also true many culturally deaf females are unaware that they need not to tolerate the treatment of sexual abuse by males (hearing or deaf).

The fear of humiliation or misplaced guilt often prevent a culturally deaf female from confronting and exposing an abuser. The problem of sexual abuse is as prevalent in the deaf culture as in any other society, but becomes much larger problem because of the communication barriers and the gossip nature of a tightly closed-knit culture such as the deaf community. This is compounded when the abuser is hearing, especially when it is a hearing person who is perceived to be a "friend of the deaf," such as an interpreter or counselor. They can take advantage of a deaf person dependent on the person. The abuser is likely to have the additional knowledge that a victim from a deaf culture is unlikely to expose her abuser.

Leaders of the culturally deaf should expose both hearing and deaf people convicted of sexual abuse instead of, as it happens more often than you would think, protecting them from further embarrassment. These abusers should be made examples of, thus discouraging others, knowing that they, too, could be made examples. More awareness and education should be provided to ensure sexual abuse is not tolerated in the deaf community. *not a mental handicap.*

easily pc deaf? Social behavior deemed acceptable and tolerated in a dormitory environment may not necessarily be accepted outside the deaf culture. Nearly everyone in the deaf community knows of members who have been tossed out of hotels and banned from public restaurants for only exhibiting "normal dorm behavior." In their defense, how does one learn proper decorum for one culture when they live in another?

Dorm life breeds a different mind set in a person. In the dorm, your friends become your family and it is carried over into adult life. While not necessarily a bad thing in itself, there seems to be noted difficulty for them to establish a "real" family relationship in marriage later in life. This is compounded when friends from the "dorm family" interfere out of a habit derived from the deaf school dormitory experience.

A deaf couple seriously attempting to start a family life will often cut themselves off from their friends in order to succeed. There does seems to be a collaboration between successful family and career-type objectives and a limitation of socialization.

To further this discussion of deaf culture "norms," lets focus on a yearly event held by and for the culturally deaf. This is a retreat, with an outdoors theme veiling its primary purpose of a social function. Its popularity often draws over a thousand deaf visitors.

While the event in itself is worthwhile as it raises funds for support services for deaf children and provides enjoyable vacations for many of the culturally deaf. However, some of the incidents occurring here and somewhat accepted as "normal" may prove to be a real eye opener for those uninitiated with the deaf community.

The event is promoted as a family type atmosphere, but at the same time they have an "everybody's welcome" policy. This consequentially causes the exposure of the many children to illegal and immoral behavior by adults such as public drunkenness, lewd behavior and drug dealings and usage. (In one case, a well-known, deaf medical-school graduate was found to be dealing drugs to 11 year-old children at the event.)

While some organizers of the event did attempt to rectify the situation, others seemed to be more concerned with "offending" them and getting the event harmed with the reputation of being "strict."

There were also three rapes reported to the county sheriff's office that week. Obviously, not all the culturally deaf people behave like this, but they are unwilling to establish proper decorum for those who need it and police themselves. Too many people were just caught up in the enjoyment of the festivities not realizing the exposure of the children to their behavior.

Among the culturally deaf is the seemingly casualness towards sexual abuse. In one instance at the retreat, I saw two culturally deaf teenagers, in their late teens, talking. They were standing by the beach watching a young culturally deaf mother and her three children wade in the lake. The mother was wearing a swimsuit and the subject of their conversation.

At one point, one signed to the other, in clear view of all the deaf people and children in the area, "I wish to rape that woman." He didn't say he was fantasizing about wanting to have sex with that girl. He wanted to *rape* her. The two continued their conversation in a casual manner as I turned to the husband that didn't see them and explained what I saw.

He confronted them and told them that he was the woman's husband. They both quietly slithered away and although the husband kept an eye out for them, it was the end of the matter.

It is, unfortunately, common and typical for such an incident like this to occur and have nothing much done about it. It seems to me in a normal society this would be reported and the scoundrels rounded up, exposed and banished from the events, if not criminal action taken against them. The two young men behaved the way they did because the deaf culture as it is today, lets them get away with it.

There seems to be a huge lack of awareness among the culturally deaf of our society's acceptance and tradition of a gratuity for certain services performed. Taxi drivers, bellhops, porters, maitr'd and the like are rarely tipped by the deaf community. Waitresses are grossly under-tipped if a gratuity is left at all. They are ignorant to the fact waitresses need the tips to offset their traditionally low wages. The culturally deaf often feel because they are deaf, they should be on the side of receiving "handouts," not be in the position of giving it to other people who are not deaf.

One ugly incident brings to light how prevalent this is. I once attempted to enter a nationally known chain restaurant with a group of deaf people in a major cultural center of the deaf. We were barred from entry by the restaurant manager. He told me deaf people kept coming in the restaurant, sitting in the booths, many never ordering food, never leaving tips and sometimes slip out without paying the tab.

I convinced the manager to seat us as some of us were from out of town and it was not right to discriminate against a whole group of people for the actions of a few.

We were seated and served with courtesy and respect, however, right after we started to leave, all 15 deaf people (I counted) got up and left without leaving a tip for the waitresses. One couple even talked of hiding in the rest room and walk out later without paying the check. I was aghast! I rounded everybody up and steered them back to the tables and collected a reasonable tip for the waitresses. I also ensured that the couple paid their tab.

Later that night, instead of discussion on the learning experience from earlier in the day, the conversation seemed focused on my being the "bad guy" who emptied their pocketbooks at the restaurant. Every single one was a graduate of a residential school for the deaf. good pl.

This inbred expectation of handouts manifests itself in other ways. A recreational club for the deaf in a large community was fortunate to receive a large block of tickets from a national major league ball club during playoff time. It was donated with the stipulation of raising funds for the club.

experience.

It presented a excellent opportunity for the club to fill the club treasury to support more programs for the deaf community. However, some of the members and officers of the club decided they would just attend the games themselves instead of using the tickets for fundraising.

Eventually the donations were cut off, and the club reputation was tarnished before the realization of improper behavior was apparent to some of them. Others were more concerned of the loss of their privileged status in the deaf community by not being able to go to anymore "free" games. This also caused internal strife within the club thus harming an organization that was otherwise progressive in providing services for the deaf community.

Some members of the deaf community are often guilty of misplaced criticism towards hearing people interested in helping the deaf.

This most pronounced when directed at sign language interpreters. I agree with the culturally deaf there are some truly bad interpreters out there, but most of the criticism is uncalled for. The majority of them are those who got into the field having an interest in the deaf and are therefore not "natural" signers. The "natural" signers are hearing people who have deaf parents, or deaf siblings, or even sometimes deaf spouses or children and are fluent in ASL almost as if it were their natural language.

Many of the sign language interpreters for the deaf learned their skills from sign language classes (or from deaf friends or other methods) and like any other class, there are those who excel and there are those who don't. Yet, the deaf culture seems to throw a blanket of criticism towards everybody in this group. The deaf culture cannot expect exact perfection from this group. It is unfair to expect everybody in this group to master ASL. The deaf culture itself doesn't always thrive for perfection within itself, so how can it demand perfection from others?

Obviously, the deaf can expect performance guideline standards, already are in existence, to qualify competent interpreters and weed out the truly bad. However, calls for even more regulations such as requiring high-level college education for all interpreters, and at the same time complaining the costs have gotten out of hand, is not a solution. Who did they expect to pay for the interpreters' secondary education? They can't get it "free" like the deaf culture have come to expect of their own secondary education.

This is an example of the deaf culture shooting itself in the foot. The "natural" signers are a finite number. Imposing further restrictions on interpreters and subsequently discouraging future would-be interpreters, would dwindle the number in the pool at a time when many of the deaf are complaining about a lack of good interpreters.

A system of rewarding good interpreters financially will motivate them to strive for excellence. More rules and regulations without economic benefits will not produce more good interpreters.

A side point, often overlooked by the deaf culture, many of these "naturally" skilled interpreters are in the business reluctantly. By this I mean they didn't necessarily intend to be an interpreter or truly have any interest in the deaf. Economic factors and their advantage of having a skill that was in great demand lead to their being one. By contrast, "non-natural" interpreters had an interest in helping the deaf or wanting to know sign language. These people are truly more likely to be concerned of the success of the deaf.

A CHILD SACRIFICED

The deaf culture often exhibits this type of favoritism towards many hearing people working or socializing among the culturally deaf. They are more attracted to the "natural" signers among hearing people and ignoring, sometimes, those who are truly concerned for them.

Judgments of hearing people, and even deaf people, often are made in reference to their ability to sign rather than their real qualifications for their positions. The Gallaudet University protest comes to mind. Harm has been dealt to deaf people because of this.

In adult life, many of the culturally deaf will continue to support some of their misguided popular leaders on positions that may even be detrimental to themselves or other culturally deaf people, instead of taking a stand against them.

For example, a culturally deaf writer describes the critical role local clubs are to large deaf sport organizations and at hand today, action is being taken by deaf leaders potentially harming local clubs. [3]

Such a case occurred at a delegate business meeting for an adult deaf sport organization. A proposal was on the table for new rules having a side effect of harming many smaller local clubs and perhaps, even leading to their demise. However, no delegate wanted to take a position opposing a popular leader sponsoring the proposal, even if it meant harming their own club.

The measure failed that year only due to intervention by this writer. After the narrow failure of his proposal during a secret ballot, the sponsoring delegate got up, threatened me because I "ruined his plans," and stormed out of the meeting. No wonder nobody else dared to challenge this man.

A CHILD SACRIFICED

To further this in a comical manner, this man, honored for his "dedication" to the organization the previous year, gave our team of young kids a 188 to 29 point drubbing during a mismatched game in the tournament. Afterwards, he came to our players and told them he was punishing them for what I "did" to him. Leaders such as this hold many deaf people hostage. As hostages, they are careful not to "offend" those leaders.

In the following year, the same measure was again brought to the floor and this time passed in my absence. In the following years the sport organization experienced a declining number of local member clubs.

The moral here is: many leaders of the deaf cannot be depended on to provide true leadership nor they should be taken at their word of knowing what is best for the culturally deaf. While the culturally deaf will have to live with the consequences of their leaders' actions, the mainstream society should take note.

With deaf schools being smaller in relation to the large public high schools in the country, the deaf students have a decided advantage when it comes to sports. With a smaller number of students, nearly everybody can play on the team.

The downside of this is discipline. It is not as easy to replace suspended or disciplined players, thus it seems high school coaches have to spend most of the time keeping key players happy. The best players on the team often call the shots and the coaches are diminished in respect.

Sadly, the attitudes learned at the high school level is often carried into adult life as I had the misfortune of finding out first-hand. Our deaf adults sports team played in a 50-team city league one year. In spite of the fact emphasis was placed on "watching the attitudes" and just having fun, our team, over the course of the season, was penalized more "technicals" than all the other teams in the city league combined.

I am sure the league officials, game officials and the other teams were relieved when the deaf team failed to make another appearance the following season.

Picked up early in life at the deaf school, many players carry their behavior to adult life. Some of these deaf players find it a game to belittle the other players, taunt the referees and other game officials, ruining the enjoyment of the activity for others. Unfortunately, you don't see many coaches or teammates stopping it.

Interestingly, one deaf team I was involved with played in a all-deaf league and the coaches and I suspected that a key player was going to jump to a different team prior to a tournament. Since we were sponsored with money from outside our club, as a precaution, I made up a contract and had all our players sign it. This was unprecedented in the deaf community. When we received the league sign-up forms for the end-of-season tournament, all our players were legally bound to play for us. And as we expected, a certain key person quit our team at that time.

On the day of the tournament, we found the suspected player had signed with another team. He used our team to "practice" with only to switch to a "better" out-of-town team at the final tournament. The coaches and club officials of this other deaf team had made these plans to trick us earlier in the season.

None of the coaches or officers of the popular out-of-town deaf team considered our contract serious, nor did they expect anybody from the deaf community would dare to challenge them. Least of all, they did not expect anybody in the deaf community to be clever enough to take precaution to prevent them from pulling such a stunt.

I took my document to the league officials and they determined that my contract was a legal document and could be subject to a lawsuit if they did not abide by the contract. The other team was stunned. Their maneuver had backfired and exposed them for who they really were and also the player, for attempting to trick us into misusing sponsorship funds.

I had included an escape clause for the player to get out of the contract which could be triggered by payment of a large three-figured fine. This was a number I had arbitrably came up with. Our club treasury received a windfall during the tournament as well as coming in last place.

After the tournament, many culturally deaf people and other club officials said we shouldn't have "interfered" with the player and we should have "let him play where he wanted to." They also said we shouldn't have embarrassed him or the club like that. It was apparent not too many people learned much from this adventure. *As usual, more people were upset at me for "rocking the boat" (again) than wanting to see justice prevail.*

Habitual liars and rumor-mongers that a normal society would shun, are often overlooked in the deaf community. Recreational drug users and abusers, criminals, and those with questionable morals are tolerated by most of the deaf community. This is often referred to as the "deaf ghetto" by those attempting to distance themselves from these deaf people.

Like a parent protecting their child who can do no wrong, a golden opportunity to raise the standard of life in the deaf community is lost.

A CHILD SACRIFICED

A glaring example of this occurred during the height of the Gallaudet student revolt. A culturally deaf adult, educated at the deaf school and well liked, decided to take advantage of the new-found deaf awareness to fill his pocketbook.

By having a "deaf club fundraiser," he raised hundreds of dollars from the general public who were duped into believing it was a charitable event and were all too happy to help out financially. He paid off some co-horts and pocketed the rest.

Afterwards, he bragged of his success among some members of the deaf community and even received some admirations and congratulations. A history of positive peer pressure would have circumvented this event as this person would not have wanted to endanger his status in the community. But the way the deaf community is today, he can get away with it.

Of course, there are those (including yours truly) in the deaf community who would have said something to him had they known about it. But, it would not have been the right kind of peer pressure. It is only effective when the body of the community polices itself. The leaders of the deaf community must encourage usage of the power of positive peer pressure.

The deaf community's actions are sometimes peculiar and bordering on the bizarre when outside hearing law enforcement is called in to handle a deaf-to-deaf dispute. In one instance, when a restraining order was served on a deaf man, he threatened bodily harm to the person who had filed the complaint in the presence of a law enforcement officer. The officer wasn't aware of the threat as it was conducted in sign language and it never occurred to the girl being threatened to tell the police officer.

A CHILD SACRIFICED

There is a general lack of understanding of a police officer's primary concern, that being to protect the citizens. Some members of the deaf community live in needless fear by not asking for the help.

However, this is further complicated when the person in the example was eventually arrested by the police for violation of the restraining order. Rather than gather around and support the victim, many members in the community accused her of doing such a terrible thing to the popular leader by calling the police. She was placed in a position of having to abandon her deaf "family" and call in an "outsider" for her own personal protection. The unwritten rule seems to be to solve deaf-to-deaf problems "internally," where unfortunately, the justice of "popularity" seems to often prevail.

It appears that when a member of the deaf culture runs afoul of our society's laws, great strides are made to protect these people from further embarrassment and from discovery within the deaf culture. Of course, this doesn't apply to everybody or every crime.

A case in point raises the absurdity of this behavior. One well known and popular member of the deaf community had an accounting business. His clients consisted of older and elderly deaf customers. He earned their trust through his willingness to do extra services for them and providing enjoyable (and looked forward to) company for them.

Unfortunately, he also stole from some of his clients and misused credit cards entrusted to him. Many of these clients were confined to their homes and had no other easy access to services and he used this trust and vulnerability to his advantage. He had made a business of preying on the elderly. He was arrested and eventually convicted for theft and fraud.

A CHILD SACRIFICED

Many of the deaf people in the deaf community do not read newspapers, thus few read of his arrest, conviction and jail sentence. It is a unique situation where people don't know about it and those few who do are "protecting" him from further embarrassment. When I was first told of this by someone in the deaf community, I told him I was going to warn some of the elderly clients. He replied saying he made a mistake now in telling me!

The reality is that public records are open to the general public to inform society of who these people are and for society to react in taking steps to protect themselves. The deaf community is not being served when some deaf people try to "protect" these criminals from the very people they violated.

Some of these elderly senior citizens, after being told of the conviction and jail sentence, gave a sign of relief. They had previous concerns about evidence of missing cash, disappearance and later, reappearance of credit cards, and disturbed financial files leading them to wonder about their own senility and often caused strife in their own households!

Some of the educated and professional culturally deaf people in the locale where this incident occurred, generally responded it was a matter to remain unspoken, although acknowledged the behavior as disgusting.

The reason for this can be attributed to the limited number of culturally deaf people and to banish members from the culture for whatever reasons, could bring about its demise. As well as the other factor being the historical tradition of nobody wanting to "rock the boat." This person is still a popular member of the deaf community.

Many graduates of the residential deaf school are fully unprepared to work in the mainstream society, let alone search for a job. They are often unprepared for dealing with unions, knowing their rights on the job and how to function with co-workers and supervisors. They are taken advantage of, work the worst shifts, passed over for promotions, and often remain in the lower pay scales indefinitely. Fear of losing their jobs, and hesitation to deal with hearing people, encourages them to learn to be content with their plight. Others quit all too soon expecting immediate gratification in wages, shifts and working conditions. The additional factors of health and welfare benefits, retirements pension, seniority rules regarding "bumping" and "bidding" complicates the work experience.

Looking for a job consists of a lot more than filling out one application and then sitting and waiting at home. An amazing amount of culturally deaf adults do just that. When asked about their job search, a typical reply would be, "I applied at so and so company two months ago and I am waiting," at the same time complains of not being able to find work.

The reality is that most applications are screened and trashed within days and an application doesn't hand anybody a job. Looking for work is a full time job in itself, and unfortunately many potential employers quietly trash a deaf application to avoid dealing with disabled employees. There are so many other methods of getting a job nowadays that it has become a science.

More preparation towards the finding and living with a job is needed during their educational years in order to get the often naive culturally deaf graduate into becoming a taxpayer.

One thing I find that exists nearly everywhere in the deaf culture is the dislike of labor unions. I have found many of them are unable to grasp the concept of a union.

A CHILD SACRIFICED

The stumbling point seems to be the fact that the union works for *them*. Too many deaf people summarily categorize unions with management, looking at both, as "hassles" and have the wrong impressions unions are a form of "tax."

This is on the contrary as unions can ensure the deaf employees of their rights and benefits. In addition, they can handle management for them and prevent management from using them or taking advantage of their ignorance.

Some fault can be attributed to some unions not taking the time to fully explain their function or a tendency to avoid dealing with the deaf. The deaf workers need to be assertive and remember that the union works for them and the union officials have to answer to the membership of the bargaining unit.

As an acquaintance to more than a few state vocational rehabilitation counselors, it is my understanding the culturally deaf DVR clients are the least responsible, have the highest failure rate (determined by whether a case is closed by fulfillment of its objectives), and most likely to abuse benefits. Many culturally deaf people expect and demand services at the same time show little cause and responsibility to be worthy of services. They don't seem to understand the services are provided by society with the purpose of turning someone into a taxpayer, thus an investment of our society's funds, *not money due to them because they are deaf.*

Most people, whether deaf or not, have run across people peddling fingerspelling cards ("ABC cards") in the transportation centers and streets of large cities. On the back of these cards would be a description that would read something along the lines: "I am deaf and I sell these cards for a living, please give what you can." Sometimes this may be a hearing person masquerading as a deaf person, but the large majority of them are ingenious culturally deaf persons trying to fill their pockets with additional dollars. Stories of $300 dollars made in several hours is not uncommon. Very few of these beggars are truly in need since the vast majority also obtain Social Security benefits. Most of the money donated to them goes to support their recreational drug and alcohol activities.

Incidentally, this is one of the few types of activities the deaf community already frown upon which helps keeps it from being more prevalent than it already is. The leaders of the deaf community should take note how the power of peer pressure can establish the proper decorum in a culture.

In the culturally deaf world, a number of adult deaf couples will wish for deaf children and often are disappointed when they have normal kids. Often, they will favor the deaf siblings over the hearing ones.

To have deaf children is something like a status symbol in the deaf community. Other deaf people are more interested in one's children if they are deaf. For a culturally deaf couple, having deaf children provides the culturally deaf world the ultimate candidates to sustain the deaf culture and also places them in a higher tier in the deaf community social class.

A CHILD SACRIFICED

CHAPTER SIX
DEAF CULTURE CORNUCOPIA

THE DEAF CULTURE, A CREATION. Some writers, including some culturally deaf, maintain the culture was created for political purposes. The existence of this culture has been presented as fact when in reality being nothing more than speculation.

I feel this "culture" label has been used almost like a weapon by the culturally deaf leaders on the general public to ensure their world continues to thrive. Many culturally deaf writers proclaim "new discoveries," a "linguistic minority," and other hype to achieve their agenda.

There are many facts available presenting the deaf "culture" as not being a true culture. Some writers admit of their doubts of a true existence in their works on the deaf culture. I feel a more descriptive and accurate word than "culture," although humorous, is "club." 4

ASL IS A LANGUAGE CONTROVERSY. I do not in any way doubt the importance of sign language for deaf people, however, the stressing of ASL (American Sign Language) by the culturally deaf as the only language for the deaf, harms the members and furthers the gap between the mainstream society and the deaf community by the devaluation of English.

Attempts by some factors to modify ASL to conform more to English (such as Signed Exact English, and Total Communication, among others) has provoked the ire of others wanting to preserve their "language."

Despite the lack of any study showing a clear cut advantage of a strictly ASL education, and even condemnation from many leaders and educators in the deaf community, the apparent importance of preventing ASL from becoming "a lost art" seems to override the true needs of a deaf child. 5

ASL IS "BABY TALK." A backlash is occurring in some cultural centers of the deaf community against ASL. Even some of the deaf staff members at Gallaudet University feel that ASL is "baby talk," and have gone as far as criticizing residential state deaf schools for not preparing deaf kids better for the world after high school. This should further discount any claim by the deaf community of any "natural" language of the deaf.

"US" VS. "THEM" STATE OF MIND. A few leaders of the culturally deaf have gone on public record of not willing to compromise with any other organizations of deaf groups differing philosophically, for the sake of a universal unity for the deaf cause. This is in spite of numerous accounts showing alliances providing gains otherwise unobtainable.

This is further complicated by statements calling for only *deaf* people selected for *deaf*-related positions regardless of the qualifications of hearing people. A form of reverse discrimination, this the effect of having it both ways. Along with articles "wondering where hearing people fit in the deaf community?," and such, may be widening the gap from the mainstream hearing society by propitiating this "us" vs. "them" state of mind. 6

RESIDENTIAL SCHOOLS FOR THE DEAF PRESERVES THE DEAF CULTURE. Virtually undisputed by all factors, is the importance of such schools to the deaf community as the deaf culture would be non-existent without them.

As "vital link," it preserves the culture for the next generation of deaf children. Stories told in the dorm, passes the culture of a previous generation to the next. The deaf social life and language is carried on.

Closing of such schools is sternly opposed by the deaf community. Most deaf children have hearing parents and the culture cannot be passed on at "home." The deaf community has to favor residential deaf schools for better or worse.

A few leaders of the deaf community have even gone to an extreme by calling closures of such residential schools "cultural genocide." 7

COCHLEAR IMPLANTS. These miniatures electronic devices are surgically implanted in profoundly deaf candidates as a kind of rudimentary listening device. While rather experimental, they provide an alternative for those who have none. This kind of development is necessary for the further advancement of medical technology in the audiology field. In order for the implants to be highly effective on children, it usually has to be implanted pre-lingually. Thus, a dilemma for the deaf community, fired up over this device.

A CHILD SACRIFICED

Experts have called merits for the implants, "unquestionable," and at the same time, the deaf community are against the cochlear implant on early aged deaf children, *even when perfection is achieved!* This device has been often called the greatest threat to the deaf culture as it takes a deaf child out of their environment.

The leaders of the deaf community have continually challenged the Food and Drug Administration's approval of the device. Proclaiming a deaf child has a "right" to be who they are, they are asserting for non-treatment of a disability on behalf of *all* deaf children. [8]

MILITANCY IN THE DEAF COMMUNITY. Noted writers have indicated an increase of "militancy" among some members of the deaf community. They have often projected themselves as "anti-hearing" much in the same way ethic and racial groups in the past have conducted their uprisings.

"Down with English" and other slogans detrimental towards the deaf cause have provoked some leaders of the deaf community to comment on the harm being bestowed on the deaf community, while other leaders are often influenced by these cult-like groups. [9]

NO GRASP OF THE AMERICAN POLITICAL PROCESS. For one reason or another, the deaf community has shut itself out of our society's political system. Most seem to live in ignorance and very few are registered voters. Many that do vote often support the "popular" leaders who may actually detrimental to the deaf community's positions and beliefs.

A CHILD SACRIFICED

Leaders, sometimes with good intentions, are often frustrated with the seemingly lack of response or dislike of actions from political leaders, and may respond with protests demanding changes. (the Gallaudet revolt comes to mind) While protests are great for raising awareness in our society and its elected leaders, *to utilize a protest to bypass the political process is anarchy.*

AMERICAN DEAF CULTURE SUBSIDIZED WITH TAXPAYER DOLLARS. Virtually every aspect of the deaf community is dependent on governmental support in one form or another.

This starts with the publicly funded state residential and day deaf schools. There are the publicly funded deaf colleges and deaf programs in hearing colleges. Also, taxpayer supported deaf agencies and support services for the deaf. Government-supported Vocational Rehabilitation programs fund the bulk of the culturally deaf post-high school education and job trainings. This includes both the education and services provided for the deaf as well as job opportunities for the deaf in operating these schools, programs and agencies.

Entitlement programs such as the federal Social Security Disability benefits as well as Supplemental Security Income and Medicare health benefits, supports a large percentage of the deaf community. State funded public assistance (welfare), food stamps, and public health clinics are heavily utilized by the culturally deaf.

The Rehabilitation Services Administration monies for years seeded many deaf research and development programs as well as entertainment programs for the deaf, such as the National Theatre of the Deaf and Captioned Films for the Deaf as well as closed captioning on television. Also, a mental health center for the deaf, a leadership training program, and many others.

Indirectly, the deaf obtain monies and services from non-profit agencies at reduced cost. State and Federal laws mandating the availability of Telephone Devices for the Deaf, (TDD's) telephone relay services and greatly reduced long distance charges at the expense of the other non-deaf users of the nation's phone system.

The list goes on and on with inane examples such as free public transportation passes in one metropolitan area to reduced admission fees to publicly-owned facilities in another.

AMERICANS WITH DISABILITIES ACT. The ADA was long overdue and necessary legislation. However, some deaf and hearing writers alike, express concern over the way it has been enacted, some for the dislike of a "forced charity," others concerned of the undue burden on the small businessman.

I feel the deaf community does not truly grasp the importance of small businesses to our society. We are a nation of small businesses, some financially better than others.

This very issue arose in a nationally syndicated writer's column concerned of the impact on small businesses. A leader of the deaf community responded with a published statement implying the cost of accommodating deaf people should be absorbed by the small business as "necessary expense." This was said, perhaps a little too easily, by someone having been college educated at public expense and currently employed in a prominent publicly-funded position.

While large businesses and many small businesses can justifiably comply with the ADA, the reality is many companies are struggling to survive in the competitive nature of the business world, and the ADA will sink a few, not to mention those that will now fail to start up.

By demanding strict compliance to the ADA, with no accommodations from the deaf community, they are in reality *hurting the society that subsidizes them.* 10

SOCIAL SECURITY BENEFITS. Virtually every culturally deaf adult is eligible for either Social Security Disability (SSD) or Supplemental Security Income benefits (SSI). It is undisputed a large percentage of the deaf community is receiving these relatively generous benefits with no intention to ever join the public work force. Abuses of the system by many of them are legendary.

Leaders of the deaf community must accept a bulk of the responsibility for this malady. It is too acceptable in the deaf society to be receiving these benefits and it is not looked down upon as a form of "welfare" which it actually is.

Deaf community newspapers and publications actually encourage this dependency with articles on how to apply for SSD/SSI benefits as well as information on applying for other public assistance benefits.

This is an ironic contradiction as the same deaf newspapers call for higher respect and standards for deaf people. 11

DEAFNESS, A BIRTHRIGHT, NOT A DIS-ABILITY. "We are not disabled, "deafness does not need to be cured, it's our birthright." Many leaders of the deaf community proclaim of this "different way of being," as a natural right of the deaf. This rhetoric is seen constantly to reinforce an image of an existence of a deaf "culture."

However, when "disability-related" benefits are available, these same people are quick to harvest the benefit monies. The classification of "disabled" is never questioned when our government hands out taxpayer dollars to support deaf people. The deaf community was strongly behind the enacting of the Americans with *Disabilities* Act, expecting to reap years of benefits, and the leaders of the deaf community have no moral conflict on the contradiction they present to the American public.

The bold truth is the deaf community *never* questions its eligibility for disability benefits and at the same time demands not to be classified as "disabled." If the leaders of the deaf "culture" wants to be judged upon favorably by future historians, they are heading in the wrong direction. 12

WRONG CHOICES IN LIFE. The deaf community condemns any deaf person educated by the oral method. They are not accepted readily into the deaf community by having made a wrong choice in life. "Thinking like hearing" or usage of speech is often unacceptable and is viewed as a negative value by the deaf community.

The deaf community will often be cold, indifferent and pretentious towards the orally educated deaf, while at the same time, actually be more civil towards hearing people.

Generally speaking, the knowledge and skill of ASL, having attended a residential deaf school or having culturally deaf parents weighs heavily on the judgment of other deaf people than the actual degree of deafness. 13

LOWERED EXPECTATIONS. Numerous writers, both hearing and deaf, have discussed the problem of residential schools and their graduates having lowered achievement levels. While some schools seem to be better than others, the average school has "disappointing results," especially when compared to their hearing counterparts.

Aside from academic failures, there are the "moral" failures of the dormitory life and it does not help that some deaf schools have had physical and sexual abuse problems.

Defense from the deaf community comes in the form of "vital" need, protection of deaf identity and *preventing the deaf culture from extinction.* 14

MORE LOWERED EXPECTATIONS. There has been a trend by some of the leaders of the deaf community calling for lowering English standards for college-educated culturally-deaf individuals.

For example, focusing on teacher competency exams, they wish to make it easier for deaf people to be certified to teach. By claiming ASL as being the natural language of the deaf, not English, they feel deaf people should not be expected to meet the same standard as hearing teachers.

Also, by claiming to have "deaf pride" and asking deaf people to stop apologizing for their poor English skills, they are in effect asking the community not to strive for the best they can be.

Other deaf leaders have countered this with this belief a lowering of standards among teachers will contribute towards making it even more difficult for a deaf child to learn English.

If this movement becomes reality, it will even further the gap between the deaf community and the hearing world as it will be more difficult for even an "educated" deaf person to get employment in the hearing society. The image of "subpar education" may be present in employers minds whether true or not. We are already struggling to overcome the inaccurate images imbedded in our society of deaf people from past generations. 15

SHORT RANGED GOALS AND LACK OF RESPONSIBILITY. A large percentage of deaf adults and children are passive, having only immediate goals. There is also ample evidence they fail to take responsibility for themselves and their actions. This can be attributed to both, being deaf and the type of education received.

I feel this, along with the tendency of some culturally deaf people to be naive, can be circumvented with early education to eliminate this pre-disposition at a facility more in line with the hearing society than a segregated facility. 16

"GIMME" ATTITUDE. Borrowing this phrase coined by one deaf writer, and "expecting a good deal of accommodations" by another, summarize perfectly this attitude.

Because they are deaf, many feel they should be on the receiving end of handouts. Everything is given to them without them asking for it. They have come to expect it and see nothing wrong to ask to get everything and anything "free" or at reduced costs.

While some writers blame the hearing society because of a "communication problem" for this, educational programs have been developed to help control this problem.

I, for one, have been embarrassed so many times by culturally deaf people asking for "handicapped" discounts on common everyday items that even truly disabled people would never dream of asking for. 17

A CHILD SACRIFICED

DESTRUCTIVE TRAITS. While the positive attributes of a deaf community are attractive to many deaf people (mostly, the close-knit, family-like social atmosphere), there is a flip side to the same coin.

Not widely known to the outside world as the deaf community deliberately shield certain information from them, is the unfortunate prevalence of gossip, backstabbing and rumor-mongering that would be a real eye-opener to those new to the deaf community. One deaf writer classifies gossip as one of the mainstays of the deaf community. He also states many culturally-deaf people are lacking in dreams and ambition. Lowered expectations have a lot to do with this. Jealousy seems to be another reason these conditions exist.

The same writer describes the community being a "solidarity," and group loyalties has made the deaf community into a rigid conformist society. Thus, anyone trying to "rock the boat," or attempt real achievements threatens the others.

I cannot emphasize enough how widespread and infectious this is. Very little true progressive achievements can be made in the deaf community because of the excessive amount of time needed to overcome conformity.

Sadly, in the deaf community, one is more apt to be engaged in a conversation pertaining to how one is able to get more services and "benefits," than any discussion on becoming self-sustaining or how one can become a contributor to society.

Many deaf people, having lived their whole lives in the deaf community, are set back with disbelief just anybody can get up and write a book. (This book with my views, for example, brought numerous "you can't do that" responses from culturally-deaf people because the community's "rules" do not permit it.) It is further difficult for them to accept that just ordinary people can make our leaders accountable for their words and actions. This accountability applies to elected leaders in the hearing world as well. (Several members of the deaf community were stunned that a local newspaper would publish my letter-to-the-editor referring to the Mayor as being inept. Incidentally, the Mayor choose not to run for re-election.) 18

CHILDREN LOST TO THE DEAF "CULT." There are numerous accounts of hearing parents "losing" their deaf children to a separate culture. Some have stated they feel the deaf community is trying to "snatch" them and need to "protect" their deaf children from them.

The deaf community is different from the parents world and the parents mostly do "lose" the child to the deaf community. However, deaf people are free to join or leave the community at their own free will.

I feel the methods to maintain the deaf culture status quo is where the deaf leaders evoke the "cult" connection. This is a real fear, as the concern for the culture often outweighs concern for a single deaf child. 19

PARENTAL "SAVIORS." One specialist on deafness hits it right on the money of parental anxiety over the discovery of deafness in their child. Wanting to do the right thing for their child, they often find, or try to find, a "savior" knowing all the right answers and decisions. Too often, they give the role to someone who will encourage them to select their "pet" method, rather than make an objective decision based upon their unique child and family situation.

Other "specialists" may encourage parents to "accept" the fact of their child's deafness and send them away to a residential school seemingly just to washing their hands of the

94

problem. Even living in the same locale as the residential school, "day students" are often discouraged, so the child gets "used" to being away from home for future considerations.

Successes and failures in the lives of deaf children every day are determined by "blind faith" decisions by parents. [20]

ENGLISH TAUGHT AS A "SECOND" LANGUAGE FOR DEAF CHILDREN. In a controversial paper published by Gallaudet University linguists and anthropologists, advocates a bilingual education, with ASL being the primary language of instruction and English taught later.

Among the other highlights, a diminished priority for speech, (to be taught later when the child is "ready") and a dismissal of usage with "mainstreaming" as for, among other things, *"instruction is likely to be based upon English!"*

Experts opposing the paper fear of future deaf adults having been limited to ASL, angry at their parents and teachers for eliminating their choices. It also goes against the culture of the United States to be a melting pot of cultures. To not integrate a minority would be a step backward. [21]

MAINSTREAMING OPTION. A viable option for deaf children. It is generally frowned upon by the deaf community, even though experts and other culturally deaf writers acknowledge a degree of success with the method.

Mainstreaming, educating the deaf alongside the hearing, introduces the deaf to the "world at large" and other benefits a writer on the deaf culture states. Others have echoed similar advantages.

The culturally-deaf are concerned of the lack of deaf role models. Some claim it disconnects the child from their rightful "culture," and shifts funds away from residential schools. Others have admitted mainstreaming provides parents a way to avoid "lowered expectation" typical of a residential school.

The mainstream movement will be tough for the deaf community to combat. While it is not an overwhelming success, it appears to have the edge over the advantages and successes of a residential deaf school. There is the irony of the current economic problems actually benefitting deaf children with the closure of some residential deaf schools forcing mainstreaming. [22]

ORAL VS. ASL, A CENTURY OF EM-BITTERMENT. The battle between the oral method (and oral-related) and the ASL "signing" method has been well documented. Both sides are guilty of being one-sided at times in their presentations to the society at large.

Some deaf leaders in the deaf community in recent years have called the oral method "repugnant" and "our enemy," and consider speech training a matter of convenience, not a necessity. An international conference on sign language was opened by the *smashing of a hearing aid with a sledgehammer* as a symbolic gesture!

Sensible experts and specialists have come to realize there is no one method to educate all deaf children. Each method has its share of successes and failures.

One item of significance common to all factors and methods is the importance of early identification of the child's deafness. This seems to be urgent in order for the greatest degree of success, regardless of the method chosen for the child. [23]

A CHILD SACRIFICED

ABSURDITIES AND OTHER DUBIOUS OCCURRENCES. The following is a collection of questionable motives by the deaf community.

Some researchers at Gallaudet University developed a method using computers to improve speech, with effective results. When a report was published in a large daily newspaper, a well known deaf leader was quoted as calling the research wasteful, and the time and money *should have been spent on improving sign language!*

A prominent deaf researcher refers to a "loss" of a "history of solutions created for them" when a deaf child is cut off or denied access to the deaf world. This seems to be a veil to support the continual existence of the deaf culture. Deaf children deserve a much better fate than the one "history" has provided.

Deaf writers have used this rhetoric "Only the deaf can decide for other deaf, likewise, only deaf are qualified to speak on issues on their behalf." Aside from damaging relationships between the deaf and hearing, a humorous continuation to that theme goes, "...only a deaf dentist knows what is best for deaf patients, ...only deaf mechanics know what is best for deaf auto owners..."

A deaf leader in a high state-level public position with authority to determine school placement deaf children in his state, publicly brags of the percentage deaf children in his state being in a residential school as being one of the highest in the nation. I shudder to think how many deaf children in that state were sent to residential schools for the "numbers consideration" over any truly objectively made decisions on behalf of the children.

Deaf leaders often speak of some deaf people and children of certain personalities, (read non-conforming to their culture) one day "disappearing" from sight as if it was a terrible fate to have happen. This is not necessarily correct as some people have "disappeared" for the better.

A respected, and self-described totally deaf and without speech, writer and deaf educator, has belittled and diminished the value of speech and speech training throughout some of his written works. He also has strong opinions against methods pertaining to any use of speech. It seems to me such expert advice should not have been forthcoming from him directed at those of us having some residual hearing (experts place this at 95% of deaf people), with him not possibly being able to experience it.

The same writer explains of an elaborate need to segregate the deaf children from the hearing society. Later on in the same book, he writes of a need to integrate the deaf back into the hearing society. Which raises the question of why segregate at all? Unless of course, it ensures the continual existence of the deaf culture.

A much-honored and regarded female deaf instructor at Gallaudet University has been subject to verbal abuse, character assassination and even was physically assaulted by militant culturally deaf persons for simply having views contrary from those held by most leaders of the deaf community.

And finally, seemingly as a solution to combat the dubious reputation of dormitories at residential schools in the hearing society, two deaf superintendents of state residential deaf schools have called for the proper names of schools for the deaf to not include the word *residential!* 24

CHAPTER SEVEN
A BETTER FUTURE FOR DEAF CHILDREN

I feel some time in the 21st century, deafness as a human disfunction will perhaps cease to exist. All the efforts to sustain a deaf community will have been done in vain. Our society will eventually see beyond the deaf community's insistence of a "culture" and the sacrificing of deaf children to preserve the deaf community's prized "club-like" atmosphere.

It will be too much to ask of the mainstream society to continue financing a group of people deliberately wanting to remain deaf. Sadly, this is happening as we speak, as many deaf leaders are fighting to keep things the way they are. Progress to cure this disability for over 20 million Americans is being impeded by a group of some generally self-centered zealots claiming to be speaking on my behalf.

The deaf leaders today have a human defect that is not readily "cured," helping them achieve their agenda. By promoting the existence of a "culture," they hope to head off a day of reckoning.

One thing is for sure, if there is no medical need for the deaf community to continue, we cannot expect the leaders of the deaf community to acknowledge its obsolescence.

A CHILD SACRIFICED

Much of the leadership of the deaf community is guided by the fortunate deaf living in the "cultural centers" of the deaf community. They have the unique opportunity to both work and socialize with other culturally deaf people without much (if any) contact with the mainstream hearing world. Living this kind of lifestyle unfortunately does not exist for the majority of the culturally deaf and they hardly represent the true condition of the average deaf person.

Leaders of the deaf community outside the cultural centers are often judged as "backwards" and are suppressed by those in the cultural centers. The image of the deaf community projected to the hearing society often represent the view from the deaf culture centers.

Another critical point to remember is virtually all leaders of the culturally deaf, the educators, specialists, and other professionals of the culturally deaf, are in the position of having to be somewhat biased. *Since their jobs and livelihood depends on the existence of a deaf culture, many of them cannot be expected to be truly objectionable.*

I maintain the importance of our society having enough contributors to support themselves and those who are unable to do so. History tells of the tragic consequences of societies failing to do so. The deaf community today, as a whole, cannot support itself and has not taken enough action to do so. Because of that, I feel it is in no position dictate its excessive wishes upon our society.

I challenge the leaders of the deaf community to *listen to some of the cries within the deaf community!* Put a priority of producing more contributors to society and diminish the deaf community's dependence on taxpayer dollars.

A CHILD SACRIFICED

Upon accomplishing that goal, parents of deaf children may truly be able to heed the call to place their child in the deaf community's hands. Trust is earned through respect, not upon demand.

The first step in the right direction to undertake such a fundamental change in the deaf community, would be the elimination of all Social Security benefits for a hearing loss. This will give the deaf community an incentive, more than any other measure, to head in the proper direction. (not to mention raise the ire unprecedentedly in the deaf community)

Those truly in need will be served by the state welfare agencies. Pride is a big thing among many of the culturally deaf and thus many would not stoop this low if they could help it. Deaf students will still be served by state vocational rehabilitation agencies with perhaps now, a much higher incentive to succeed.

Taking a handout is too acceptable in the deaf community and change has not come from within.

The deaf can expect accommodation from the hearing world to level the playing field to offset their deafness, but after that, the deaf have to play by the same rules as everyone else.

The deaf community should be more truthful to what they truly offer to parents of deaf children. Sacrificing children to preserve the interests of a select few is asking too much. In reality, the deaf "culture" option is nothing more than another choice, for a selection, having to be made by parents based upon "which is the lessor evil?"

A CHILD SACRIFICED

REFERENCES
AND NOTES

C. Tane Akamatsu, Wilma Rose Santiago, *Deaf Life, (Does ASL Have a Place in Education for the Deaf?).* Rochester, NY: Deaf Life Press.

Lisa Allphin, *The DCARA News.* San Leandro, CA: Deaf Counseling, Advocacy and Referral Agency.

Edward Dolnick, (Sept. 1993) *The Atlantic Monthly. (Deafness as a Culture.)* Boston, MA: The Atlantic Monthly Company.

Leo M. Jacobs (1989) *A Deaf Adult Speaks Out.* Washington, D.C. Gallaudet University Press.

Henry Kisor (1990) *What's that Pig Outdoors?* New York, NY: Penguin Books.

Harlan Lane (1992) *The Mask of Benevolence.* New York, NY: Alfred A Knopf.

Jack Levesque, *The DCARA News,* San Leandro, CA: Deaf Counseling, Advocacy and Referral Agency.

David M. Luterman with Mark Ross (1991) *When Your Child is Deaf.* Parkton, MD: York Press.

A CHILD SACRIFICED

Matthew S. Moore and Linda Levitan (1992) *For Hearing People Only.* Rochester, NY: Deaf Life Press.

Carol Padden, *The Deaf Community and the Culture of Deaf People.* N/A, N/A

Carol Padden and Tom Humphries (1988) *Deaf in America, Voices from a Culture.* Cambridge, MA: Howard University Press.

Tony Papalia, *The DCARA NEWS, (Teacher Competency Tests:)* San Leandro, CA: Deaf Counseling, Advocacy and Referral Agency.

Oliver Sacks (1990) *Seeing Voices.* New York, NY: Harper-Collins Publishers.

Debra J. Saunders (1993) *San Francisco Chronicle, (Disabilities Act written so badly, it is dangerous.)* San Francisco, CA

David A. Stewart (1991) *Deaf Sport.* Washington, D.C: Gallaudet University Press.

Larry G. Stewart (1992) *A Deaf American Monograph, Viewpoints on Deafness, (Debunking the Bilingual/Bicultural Snow Job in the American Deaf Community.)* Silver Springs, MD: National Association of the Deaf.

RECOMMENDED FURTHER READING:

On the direction headed by the deaf culture-*"Debunking the Bilingual/Bicultural Snow Job,"* by Larry G. Stewart.

For objective information on deafness in children-*"When Your Child is Deaf,"* by David M. Luterman with Mark Ross.

A CHILD SACRIFICED

PERTINENT INFORMATION REGARDING THE NOTES SECTION:
The information in the notes section is provided as a source of further information for the reader and compliance with the U.S. Copyright laws regarding "fair use." The reader should not assume the positions on any subject matter of the source authors in the notes section without having read their actual writings. Those authors may, or may not, have been citing the positions of others, quoting others or simply engaged in a general discussion of the subject.

1. Padden and Humphries, pg. 2, L. Stewart, pg. 135.
2. Jacobs, pg. (back cover).
3. D. Stewart, pg. 13.
4. L. Stewart, pg. 129.
5. Luterman, ("lack of clear cut advantage") pg. 145, Padden and Humphries, ("a lost art") pg. 60, L. Stewart, pg. 132-133, Akamatsu and Santiago, pg. 31.
6. Lane, ("alliances providing gains") pg. 22, Levesque, ("not willing to compromise") April-May, 1990, ("only deaf in deaf-related positions") March, 1988, October, 1987, L. Stewart, ("us vs. them") pg. 134.
7. Allphin, October, 1992, January, 1992, Lane, pg. 13, 107, Moore and Levitan, pg. 101, Padden and Humphries, pg. 6, Sacks, Pg. 60, 138.
8. Kisor, pg. 239, Lane, ("greatest threat to deaf community," also, "even when perfection is achieved") pg. 26, 236-237, Levesque, ("right to be who they are") June-July 1992, (also, a rebuttal to a "letter to the editor,") August, 1992), Luterman, ("unquestionably") pg. 122.
9. Kisor, pg. 145, 160-161, Luterman, pg. 20, L. Stewart, pg. 129.
10. DCARA News, ("necessary expenses") April, 1993, Kisor, ("forced charity") pg. 263, Saunders, (syndicated writer) January 15, 1993.
11. DCARA News, April, 1992, pg 13.
12. Lane, pg. 21, Levesque, June-July, 1992, L. Stewart, pg. 134-135.
13. Lane, pg. 5-6, 17, Luterman, pg. 156, Padden, pg. 98, Padden and Humphries, pg. 51, 54.
14. Moore and Levitan, pg. 101.
15. Levesque, April, 1992, April, 1993, Papalia, January, 1991, pg. 5, L. Stewart, pg. 135.

A CHILD SACRIFICED

16. Jacobs, ("short-ranged goals") pg. 81, Luterman, ("passive, fails to take responsibility") pg. 30-31.
17. Jacobs, ("gimme") pg. 82-88, Kisor, ("accommodations") pg. 265, Padden and Humphries, pg. 43-44.
18. Moore and Levitan, pg. 213-215.
19. Luterman, pg, 21, 151, Sacks, pg. 119-120.
20. Jacobs, ("used to being away from home") pg. 2, Kisor, ("send them away") pg. 21, Luterman, ("savior") pg. 38.
21. Jacobs, ("speech taught later") pg. 127, Lane, ("based on English") pg. 184, Luterman, ("angry," also, "against culture") pg. 150.
22. Kisor, pg. 32, Moore and Levitan, ("similar advantages") pg. 214, Padden and Humphries, ("shift funds away") pg. 115-116, L. Stewart, ("degree of success") pg. 133, Sacks, ("world-at-large") pg. 138.
23. Jacobs, pg. 6, ("convenience") 21, 77, ("repugnant") 112, Kisor, pg. 8, 41, 239, 254, Lane, ("sledgehammer") pg. 81, Luterman, ("no one method to educate the deaf") pg. 140, 144, 148, Padden and Humphries, ("our enemy") pg. 51, Sacks, pg. 2.
24. Allphin, ("percentage of deaf children in residential schools") March-April, 1993, Jacobs, ("disappeared") pg. 42, ("segregate-integrate") pg. 57-58, Kisor, ("researchers at Gallaudet") pg, 257, Luterman, ("95% with residual hearing") pg. 144, Moore and Levitan, ("proper name for residential schools") pg. 102, Padden and Humphries, ("history of solutions") pg. 120, L. Stewart, ("only the deaf is qualified") pg. 135, Dolnick, ("physically assaulted") pg. 52-53.

INDEX

A CHILD SACRIFICED

A CHILD SACRIFICED

to the Deaf Culture

TO ORDER A COPY FOR YOURSELF OR A FRIEND,
USE THIS HANDY ORDER FORM OR WRITE TO:

KODIAK MEDIA GROUP
PO BOX 1029-J
WILSONVILLE, OREGON 97070

QUANTITY	PRICE	SHIPPING/HANDLING	TOTAL
Single copy	$18.95	$3.95 (foreign $5.95)	$22.90
2 copies	$37.90	$3.95 (foreign $7.95)	$41.85
3 copies	$56.85	$3.95 (foreign $9.95)	$60.80

MAKE CHECK OR MONEY ORDER PAYABLE TO:
KODIAK MEDIA GROUP

RUSH ORDERS MAILED WITHIN 5 BUSINESS DAYS, ADD $2.00 PER BOOK.
CONTACT PUBLISHER FOR SPECIAL QUANTITY DISCOUNTS.
FOREIGN ORDERS, PLEASE SEND MONEY ORDER IN U.S. FUNDS ONLY.
DEALER/WHOLESALER BULLETIN AVAILABLE.

PLEASE PRINT CLEARLY!

NAME_____

ADDRESS_____

CITY_____

STATE_____ ZIP_____ PH.(____)_____